INTEGRATIVE MEDICINE
AND THE HEALTH OF
THE PUBLIC

A SUMMARY OF THE FEBRUARY 2009 SUMMIT

Andrea M. Schultz, Samantha M. Chao,
and J. Michael McGinnis, *Rapporteurs*

INSTITUTE OF MEDICINE
OF THE NATIONAL ACADEMIES

THE NATIONAL ACADEMIES PRESS
Washington, D.C.
www.nap.edu

THE NATIONAL ACADEMIES PRESS • 500 Fifth Street, N.W. • Washington, DC 20001

NOTICE: The project that is the subject of this report was approved by the Governing Board of the National Research Council, whose members are drawn from the councils of the National Academy of Sciences, the National Academy of Engineering, and the Institute of Medicine. The members of the committee responsible for the report were chosen for their special competences and with regard for appropriate balance.

Support for this project was provided by the National Academies. Any opinions, findings, conclusions, or recommendations expressed in this publication are those of the author(s) and do not necessarily reflect the views of the organizations or agencies that provided support for the project.

International Standard Book Number-13: 978-0309-13901-4
International Standard Book Number-10: 0-309-13901-5

Additional copies of this report are available from the National Academies Press, 500 Fifth Street, N.W., Lockbox 285, Washington, DC 20055; (800) 624-6242 or (202) 334-3313 (in the Washington metropolitan area); Internet, http://www.nap.edu.

For more information about the Institute of Medicine, visit the IOM home page at: **www.iom.edu.**

The serpent has been a symbol of long life, healing, and knowledge among almost all cultures and religions since the beginning of recorded history. The serpent adopted as a logotype by the Institute of Medicine is a relief carving from ancient Greece, now held by the Staatliche Museen in Berlin.

Suggested citation: IOM (Institute of Medicine). 2009. *Integrative medicine and the health of the public: A summary of the February 2009 summit.* Washington, DC: The National Academies Press.

"Knowing is not enough; we must apply.
Willing is not enough; we must do."
—Goethe

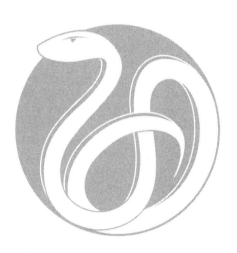

INSTITUTE OF MEDICINE

OF THE NATIONAL ACADEMIES

Advising the Nation. Improving Health.

THE NATIONAL ACADEMIES
Advisers to the Nation on Science, Engineering, and Medicine

The **National Academy of Sciences** is a private, nonprofit, self-perpetuating society of distinguished scholars engaged in scientific and engineering research, dedicated to the furtherance of science and technology and to their use for the general welfare. Upon the authority of the charter granted to it by the Congress in 1863, the Academy has a mandate that requires it to advise the federal government on scientific and technical matters. Dr. Ralph J. Cicerone is president of the National Academy of Sciences.

The **National Academy of Engineering** was established in 1964, under the charter of the National Academy of Sciences, as a parallel organization of outstanding engineers. It is autonomous in its administration and in the selection of its members, sharing with the National Academy of Sciences the responsibility for advising the federal government. The National Academy of Engineering also sponsors engineering programs aimed at meeting national needs, encourages education and research, and recognizes the superior achievements of engineers. Dr. Charles M. Vest is president of the National Academy of Engineering.

The **Institute of Medicine** was established in 1970 by the National Academy of Sciences to secure the services of eminent members of appropriate professions in the examination of policy matters pertaining to the health of the public. The Institute acts under the responsibility given to the National Academy of Sciences by its congressional charter to be an adviser to the federal government and, upon its own initiative, to identify issues of medical care, research, and education. Dr. Harvey V. Fineberg is president of the Institute of Medicine.

The **National Research Council** was organized by the National Academy of Sciences in 1916 to associate the broad community of science and technology with the Academy's purposes of furthering knowledge and advising the federal government. Functioning in accordance with general policies determined by the Academy, the Council has become the principal operating agency of both the National Academy of Sciences and the National Academy of Engineering in providing services to the government, the public, and the scientific and engineering communities. The Council is administered jointly by both Academies and the Institute of Medicine. Dr. Ralph J. Cicerone and Dr. Charles M. Vest are chair and vice chair, respectively, of the National Research Council.

www.national-academies.org

PLANNING COMMITTEE FOR THE
SUMMIT ON INTEGRATIVE MEDICINE
AND THE HEALTH OF THE PUBLIC[1]

RALPH SNYDERMAN *(Chair)*, Duke University
CAROL M. BLACK, Academy of Medical Royal Colleges
CYRIL CHANTLER, The King's Fund
ELIZABETH A. GOLDBLATT, Academic Consortium for
    Complementary and Alternative Health Care
ERMINIA GUARNERI, Scripps Center for Integrative Medicine
MICHAEL M. E. JOHNS, Emory University
RICHARD P. LIFTON, Yale University School of Medicine
BRUCE S. McEWEN, The Rockefeller University
DEAN ORNISH, Preventive Medicine Research Institute and University
    of California, San Francisco
VICTOR S. SIERPINA, University of Texas Medical Branch
ESTHER M. STERNBERG, National Institute of Mental Health
ELLEN L. STOVALL, National Coalition for Cancer Survivorship
REED V. TUCKSON, UnitedHealth Group
SEAN TUNIS, Center for Medical Technology Policy

Study Staff

JUDITH A. SALERNO, Executive Officer
J. MICHAEL McGINNIS, Senior Scholar
SAMANTHA M. CHAO, Program Officer (through February 2009)
ANDREA M. SCHULTZ, Associate Program Officer (from December
    2008)
KATHARINE BOTHNER, Research Associate (from December 2008)
JOI WASHINGTON, Senior Program Assistant
CATHERINE ZWEIG, Senior Program Assistant

---

[1] The role of the planning committee was limited to planning and preparation of the summit. This document was prepared by rapporteurs as a factual summary of what was presented and discussed at the summit.

v

Reviewers

This report has been reviewed in draft form by individuals chosen for their diverse perspectives and technical expertise, in accordance with procedures approved by the National Research Council's Review Committee. The purpose of this independent review is to provide candid and critical comments that will assist the institution in making its published report as sound as possible and to ensure that the report meets institutional standards for objectivity, evidence, and responsiveness to the study charge. The review comments and draft manuscript remain confidential to protect the integrity of the process. We wish to thank the following individuals for their review of this report:

Brent A. Bauer, Mayo Clinic
Susan Frampton, Planetree
Michael M.E. Johns, Emory University
Bruce McEwen, Harold and Margaret Milliken Hatch
　　Laboratory of Neuroendocrinology, The Rockefeller University

Although the reviewers listed above have provided many constructive comments and suggestions, they were not asked to endorse the conclusions or recommendations nor did they see the final draft of the report before its release. The review of this report was overseen by **Ada Sue Hinshaw,** Uniformed Services University of the Health. Appointed by the National Research Council and Institute of Medicine, she was responsible for making certain that an independent examination of this report was carried out in accordance with institutional procedures and that all review comments were carefully considered. Responsibility for the final content of this report rests entirely with the authoring committee and the institution.

Foreword

Health is a personal matter, as is the way each of us chooses to integrate concerns about health into our lives. Like a Rorschach blot, the notion of integrative medicine, or integrative health, means different things to different people. As an approach to enhancing health, integrative health seeks to combine the best scientific and evidence-based approaches to care with a focus on the full range of needs of the individual. Integrative medicine seeks to enable everyone to maintain their health insofar as possible, and to be empowered in partnering with health care providers when illness occurs. With this approach, patients can be more effective stewards of their own health and wellness.

This publication, *Integrative Medicine and the Health of the Public: A Summary of the 2009 Summit*, provides an account of the discussion and presentations of the two-and-a-half day summit in Washington, DC, held February 25–27, 2009. While this summary captures the discussion, it cannot adequately convey the energy and enthusiasm of the participants who filled the auditorium throughout the event. The Institute of Medicine (IOM) was honored to host such a large and diverse group to discuss such a timely topic, especially at such a critical time in American health care policy making.

Under the direction of Ralph Snyderman, the summit planning committee assembled an outstanding group of speakers and discussants who provided valuable insights on the potential and limitations of integrative health care, models that might be most conducive to its delivery, the multiple dimensions of scientific endeavor that intersect as its support base, and possible economic implications and incentives. Participants had an exceptional opportunity to examine the role and value of integrative medicine in meeting health needs and overcoming fragmentation in the health care delivery system.

The summit discussions were fruitful and collaborative, and I believe that every participant came away from the meeting having learned something each did not know before. It is my hope that this publication will advance thoughtful consideration of integrative medicine and extend the enthusiasm that was ignited at the summit.

I would like to thank the Bravewell Collaborative for their spirit of partnership and support of this activity, Ralph Snyderman for his leadership and guidance, the planning committee for their commitment and wisdom, and the IOM staff for their hard work and dedication.

Harvey V. Fineberg, M.D., Ph.D.
President, Institute of Medicine

Preface

"Life, liberty, and the pursuit of happiness," a phrase taken directly from the Declaration of Independence, indicates *the* basic values identified by the founders of our nation. Of the three, life is the most fundamental as without it, liberty and the pursuit of happiness are meaningless. Health, of course, is the underpinning of life and therefore, it is puzzling that there is so little general demand for an explicit public emphasis on nourishing health as a personal and social resource. Indeed, despite spending enough on "health care" to threaten our economy, our country is rife with chronic disease, is facing a growing epidemic of obesity and ill health, has a system of care that focuses on the treatment of episodes of disease rather than promoting health or coherently treating disease when it occurs, and there are 47 million Americans without health insurance.

It is well recognized that our approach to health care is reactive, sporadic, uncoordinated, and very expensive. Clearly, we are capable of far better health care delivery and more innovative approaches toward improving the health and well-being of our citizens. The concept of the Summit on Integrative Medicine and the Health of the Public arose from these basic premises that health and well-being represent our most valued assets and that our current delivery system is deeply flawed in its capacity to safeguard those assets. To improve health, we must address not only health care delivery but also how to engage and inform the patient (person), so they effectively achieve better health. Indeed, there are models and examples of more coherent approaches to enhancing health and well-being and preventing and caring for chronic disease. Critical to such approaches is the integration of the best of conventional care with the full engagement of an informed patient along with coordination of those therapies and services shown to improve outcomes. Thus, integration of health care to include a full range of capabilities for enhancement of health and wellness, prediction and prevention of chronic disease, as well as participation by the patient form a common theme for ways to address our current health dilemma.

These are concepts well recognized and supported by the members of the Bravewell Collaborative, a philanthropic organization committed to improving health through integrative approaches. Through a long-standing friendship with the leadership of this organization, particularly Christy Mack and Diane Neimann, we discussed how their organization could best further their agenda to improve health and well-being through integrative care. I suggested they contact the Institute of Medicine (IOM), our nation's most respected organization regarding the evaluation of health care issues. As a result of their deliberations with IOM President Dr. Harvey Fineberg and the IOM leadership, the IOM agreed to sponsor a major national summit bringing together broad program, scientific, and policy experts to review the issues and state of the science for integrative health and health care, and to discuss the feasibility of various existing models or new models as potential solutions to our current problems. The intent of summit organizers was to organize an event that offered a venue for a diverse group of stakeholders to come together for candid discussion of topics related to integrative medicine and the advancement of the field; the summit was not designed to elicit a consensus or a set of recommendations from the participants or the planning committee.

The IOM assembled a highly experienced and knowledgeable planning committee, which I was privileged to chair, and we launched a year of intensive work. None of us likely anticipated fully the time commitment involved, but for each of us the effort was a work of love. Along with support from the superb staff of the Institute of Medicine, particularly Dr. Michael McGinnis, Samantha Chao, and Andrea Schultz, we were able to assemble the program for the February 25–27 meeting described in this summary. We hoped for an audience of up to 500, but once the summit was announced, over 700 people registered, and we were able to accommodate about 600. The speakers and participants included a broad array of leaders in multiple fields. The audience, likewise, was outstanding and participated fully and effectively.

The summit not only far exceeded our highest expectations, it was an event that led to the bonding of attendees, informed our outlook, and enhanced our commitment to work for positive change. During multiple discussion venues, many facets of integrative care were explored. Of course, no single approach could be identified as *the* solution, but it was broadly agreed that health and health care must be centered on the needs of the individual throughout his or her life, supporting the individual's capability to improve health and well-being, to predict and prevent chronic disease, and to treat it effectively and coherently when it occurs. Approaches to care must be evidence based, yet caring and compassionate. Fortunately, many such integrative approaches already exist on which demonstration projects might be built to identify and validate the best integrative solutions to the various health care delivery needs.

This publication captures many of the deliberations and suggestions offered by participants as to possible next steps. As such it can be used as a touchstone not only for the meeting participants energized by their experience, but by others far beyond the meeting who are likewise committed to transformative change on behalf of better health. What better purpose to drive the focus of our attention on the path for rational attention to health care reform that cultivates health as a value for each of us and for society?

Ralph Snyderman, M.D.
Chair, Planning Committee
for the Summit On Integrative Medicine
and the Health of the Public
July 10, 2009

Acknowledgments

This publication is the product of the efforts of many individuals, and the Institute of Medicine (IOM) is grateful to all who contributed to the success of the summit.

Recognition must first go to the Bravewell Collaborative, which made the summit possible through its generous funding and its vision to integrate health and healing into the practice of medicine.

The commitment and wisdom of the members of the summit planning committee must be acknowledged. With Ralph Snyderman's leadership as chair, the planning committee assembled an agenda of distinguished speakers, whose presentations informed and inspired everyone. Thanks are also owed to the authors of the papers commissioned by the IOM, which provided background for the discussions.

Throughout the course of the project, several dedicated staff members supported the planning and execution of the summit. Andrea Schultz and Samantha Chao provided steadfast support to the planning committee and project, while Michael McGinnis and Judith Salerno offered their guidance and leadership. Thanks go to Katharine Bothner for her research assistance; to Joi Washington, Judy Estep, and Catherine Zweig for their administrative support; and to Cindy Mitchell for her incredible support to the contributions of the summit chair. Considerable appreciation is also given to Donna Duncan, Michael Hamilton, and Zimika Stewart for skillfully managing the summit logistics.

Additional thanks go to the numerous IOM staff members who contributed to the execution of the summit and to the production and dissemination of this publication: Clyde Behney, Christie Bell, Savannah Briscoe, Patrick Burke, Jody Evans, Dorea Ferris, Bronwyn Schrecker Jamrok, Abbey Meltzer, Patsy Powell, Marty Perreault, Autumn Rose,

Christine Stencel, Janet Stoll, Ariel Suarez, Vilija Teel, Lauren Tobias, Jackie Turner, Ellen Urbanski, Danitza Valdivia, Julie Wiltshire, Sarah Widner, and Jordan Wyndelts.

Finally, the insight and enthusiasm contributed by each individual who attended the three-day summit also must be recognized. The success of the summit would not have been so great without each attendee's active participation.

Contents

Table, Figures, and Boxes

TABLE

FIGURES

BOXES

Summary

On February 25–27, 2009, the Institute of Medicine (IOM) convened the Summit on Integrative Medicine and the Health of the Public in Washington, DC. The summit brought together more than 600 scientists, academic leaders, policy experts, health practitioners, advocates, and other participants from many disciplines to examine the practice of integrative medicine, its scientific basis, and its potential for improving health. This publication summarizes the background, presentations, and discussions that occurred during the summit.

INTRODUCTION

The last century witnessed dramatic changes in the practice of health care, and coming decades promise advances that were not imaginable even in the relatively recent past. Science and technology continue to offer new insights into disease pathways and treatments, as well as mechanisms of protecting health and preventing disease. Genomics and proteomics are bringing personalized risk assessment, prevention, and treatment options within reach; health information technology is expediting the collection and analysis of large amounts of data that can lead to improved care; and many disciplines are contributing to a broadening understanding of the complex interplay among biology, environment, behavior, and socioeconomic factors that shape health and wellness.

Although medical advances have saved and improved the lives of millions, much of medicine and health care have primarily focused on addressing immediate events of disease and injury, generally neglecting underlying socioeconomic factors, including employment, education, and income, and behavioral risk factors. These factors, and others, impact health status, accentuate disparities, and can lead to costly, preventable diseases (IOM, 2001b). Furthermore, the disease-driven approach to medicine and health care has resulted in a fragmented, specialized health system in which care is typically reactive and episodic, as well as often inefficient and impersonal (IOM, 2007b; Snyderman and Williams, 2003).

In health terms, the consequences of this fragmentation can be serious. Chronic conditions now represent the major challenge to the U.S. health care system. Five chronic conditions—diabetes, heart disease, asthma, high blood pressure, and depression—account for more than half of all U.S. health expenditures (Druss et al., 2001). Among Medicare recipients, 20 percent live with five or more chronic conditions and their care accounts for two-thirds of all Medicare expenditures (Anderson, 2005). Many of these conditions are preventable, but only about 55 percent of the most recommended clinical preventive services are actually delivered (McGlynn et al., 2003).

Care coordination that emphasizes wellness and prevention, a hallmark of integrative medicine, is a major and growing need for people both with and without chronic diseases. Those with chronic diseases rarely receive the full support they need to achieve maximum benefit. A patient's course of care may require contact with clinicians and caregivers and may require many transitions, for example from hospital to home care. However, these transitions often are poorly handled, leading to adverse events that result in rehospitalizations 20 percent of the time (Forster et al., 2003). The IOM report *To Err is Human* concluded that half of all adverse events are caused by preventable medical errors. Indeed, it estimated that medical errors are responsible for some 44,000 to 98,000 deaths per year, ranking errors among the nation's leading causes of death (IOM, 1999).

Disconnected and uncoordinated care amplifies the economic burden of the health care system. The costs of U.S. health care are driven in large part by the inefficiencies, redundancies, and excesses of the current fragmented system and are considered by many economists and policy makers to be unsustainable, either for individuals or for the nation. In 2009, nearly $2.5 trillion will be spent in the United States in a health care system that is underperforming on many dimensions. The current trend will drive expenditures to $4.3 trillion by 2017 (Keehan et al., 2008) unless changes are made. Despite per capita expenditures that are at least twice as high as the average for other Western nations, the United

States ranks far down the global list in the health of its citizens (Schoen et al., 2006). Estimates by various experts suggest that one-third to one-half of U.S. health expenditures do little to improve health (U.S. Congress, 2004; U.S. Congress, 2006).

Combined, economic challenges and dissatisfaction with the current system drive interest in health reforms that would offer lower-cost, more effective, holistic, evidence-based approaches. This interest is growing concurrent with, and fueled by, growth in the science base about the relationships among health, the pace of healing, and more intangible elements of the caring process, including empowerment of patients to play a central role in their care. Evidence is accumulating about the variety of factors that have important effects on health care outcomes: the interaction between an individual's social, economic, psychological, and physical environments, and his or her biological susceptibility to illness and responsiveness to treatment; the nature of the care *process*, as well as its *content*; and the often greater health benefit to be had from certain "lower tech" interventions, rather than more costly approaches.

In addition, the interest in unconventional approaches to prevention and treatment has grown. In 2007, nearly two of every five Americans over the age of 18 reported use of therapies such as yoga, massage, meditation, and natural products and supplements (Barnes et al., 2008). In total, such approaches accounted for $34 billion in out-of-pocket expenditures in 2007 (Nahin et al., 2009). And, more than half of all Americans over the age of 18 report regular use of dietary supplements, supporting a $23 billion industry (National Institutes of Health, 2006). Some of these practices are based on the experience of cultures over time, some are based on evolving scientific theories, and some are based on little more than belief. Each compels an assessment of what is lacking in conventional health care that causes so many people to turn elsewhere for help. Stakeholders must determine which models and approaches to health care, conventional or otherwise, might best integrate the science, caring, efficiency, and results that patients desire and that improve optimal health and well-being throughout the life span.

This is the background to the IOM's Summit on Integrative Medicine and the Health of the Public. Integrative medicine may be described as orienting the health care process to create a seamless engagement by patients and caregivers of the full range of physical, psychological, social, preventive, and therapeutic factors known to be effective and necessary for the achievement of optimal health throughout the life span. The aim of the meeting was to explore opportunities, challenges, and models for a more integrative approach to health and medicine. This approach could shift the focus of the health care system toward efficient, evidence-based practice, prevention, wellness, and patient-centered care, creating a more personalized, predictive, and participatory health care experience.

THE SUMMIT ON INTEGRATIVE MEDICINE
AND THE HEALTH OF THE PUBLIC

The IOM Summit on Integrative Medicine and the Health of the Public was sponsored by the Bravewell Collaborative, and was planned by a 14-member committee, chaired by Dr. Ralph Snyderman.[1] The summit was designed to consider how integrative concepts can fit within a number of initiatives for transforming the health care system, including patient-centered care; personalized, predictive, preventive, participatory medicine; mind-body relationships; the expanding science base in genomics, proteomics, and other fields; health care financing reform; shared decision making; value-driven health care; and team-based care processes.

The agenda was divided into five half-day sessions, each with a keynote speaker, a panel of expert presenters, and audience discussion. The plenary sessions covered overarching visions for integrative medicine, models of care, workforce and education needs, and economic and policy implications. One of the planning committee's goals was to afford abundant opportunity to hear from summit participants. Ample time was allowed for questions and answers during plenary sessions; luncheon discussion groups allowed participants to continue plenary discussions; and five small assessment groups discussed priorities in assigned topic areas and reported to the plenary on their discussions.

SUMMIT THEMES

The summit provided the opportunity for all attendees to hear from and provide a rich array of experiences, diverse perspectives, and a variety of fresh ideas. Certain refrains were often repeated in different ways throughout the course of the summit (see Box S-1).

---

[1]The role of the planning committee was limited to planning and preparation of the summit. This document was prepared by rapporteurs as a factual summary of what was presented and discussed at the summit.

BOX S-1
Recurring Summit Perspectives on Integrative Medicine

- **Vision of optimal health:** *alignment of individuals and their health care for optimal health and healing across a full life span*
- **Conceptually inclusive:** *seamless engagement of the full range of established health factors—physical, psychological, social, preventive, and therapeutic*
- **Lifespan horizon:** *integration across the lifespan to include personal, predictive, preventive, and participatory care*
- **Person-centered:** *integration around, and within, each person*
- **Prevention-oriented:** *prevention and disease minimization as the foundation of integrative health care*
- **Team-based:** *care as a team activity, with the patient as a central team member*
- **Care integration:** *seamless integration of the care processes, across caregivers and institutions*
- **Caring integration:** *person- and relationship-centered care*
- **Science integration:** *integration across scientific disciplines, and scientific processes that cross domains*
- **Integration of approach:** *integration across approaches to care—e.g., conventional, traditional, alternative, complementary—as the evidence supports*
- **Policy opportunities:** *emphasis on outcomes, elevation of patient insights, consideration of family and social factors, inclusion of team care and supportive follow-up, and contributions to the learning process*

These themes represent some of the characteristics and priorities coursing throughout summit presentations and participant discussions:

- **Vision of optimal health.** Integrative medicine, or integrative health care, seeks the *alignment of individuals and their health care for optimal health and healing across the life span.*
- **Conceptually inclusive.** Integrative health care means different things to different people, but common elements describe a care process in which patients and caregivers work together to foster *seamless engagement of the full range of health factors— physical, psychological, social, preventive, and therapeutic—* known to be effective and necessary to achieve optimal lifelong health.
- **Lifespan horizon.** The perspective of integrative *health care extends across the life span.* Fundamental to its philosophy is the

notion of starting as early as possible—even before birth—to plan and shape a person's health future. It is *personal, predictive, preventive, and participatory.*

- **Person-centered.** The orientation of *health care is integrated around, and within, each person.* That is, care not only accounts for differences in individual conditions, needs, and circumstances, but it also engages patients as partners in addressing the different biological, psychological, spiritual, and social and economic reference points that shape patients' wellness, illness, and healing. The intensity of care and the support mobilized are tailored to the intensity of the person's need and risk, as moderated by personal preferences.

- **Prevention-oriented.** With its focus on optimal health, *prevention and disease minimization represent the foundation of integrative health care.* The first priority for a health care system that uses an integrative approach is, therefore, to ensure that the full spectrum of prevention opportunities—clinical, behavioral, social, and environmental—are included in the care delivery process.

- **Team-based.** Integrative health care envisions *a care process that is a team activity, with the patient as a central team member.* This differs from prevailing patterns of care that are often compartmentalized, fragmented, and delayed. An integrated health team would employ professionals with a wide spectrum of expertise and skills and diverse, interdisciplinary education and training in a set of core competencies.

- **Care integration.** In integrative health care, the *seamless integration of the care processes, across caregivers and across institutions,* is the most fundamental organizational principle. Whether through the use of patient navigators or health coaches, whether through care support tools and electronic health records that support the patient focus, or whether through payment systems pegged to patient outcomes, every aspect of system design should further the goal of integration.

- **Caring integration.** *Person-centered care is also relationship-centered care.* In integrative health care, care is integrated not only across organized caregiver sites, but across the relevant life dimensions—embracing and including home, family, loved ones, and the community. Care also considers the social and economic factors that affect health, including employment status, education, income, social networks, and family support.

- **Science integration.** Integrative health care is *derived from lessons integrated across scientific disciplines, and it requires scientific processes that cross domains.* The most important influences on health, for individuals and society, are not the factors at play within any single domain—genetics, behavior, social or economic circumstances, physical environment, health care—but the dynamics and synergies across domains. Research tends to examine these influences in isolation, which can distort interpretation of the results and hinder application of results. The most value will come from broader, systems-level approaches and redesign of research strategies and methodologies.

- **Integration of approaches.** Integrative health care is *integrated across approaches to care—e.g., conventional, traditional, alternative, complementary—as the evidence supports.* In addition to the best application of conventional allopathic approaches, it may use evidence-based interventions or practices derived from ancient folk practices, cultural-specific sources, contemporary product development, or crafted from a blend of these. Sound practice requires that the standards of evidence be appropriate to the modality assessed, consistent across the range of options, and structured to assess broad outcomes over time.

- **Policy opportunities.** Policies that encourage integrative health care would define value in terms that *emphasize outcomes, elevate patient insights, account for family and social factors, encourage team care, provide supportive follow-up, and contribute to the learning process.*

In addition to these recurring themes, participants offered a number of suggestions throughout the course of the presentations, discussions, and breakout sessions on ways in which the science, practice, application, and effectiveness of integrative health and medicine might be enhanced. Specific participant suggestions and proposals included those related to:

- *Research,* such as clarification of the nature and pathways by which biological predispositions and responses interact with social and environmental influences, redesign of study protocols to better accommodate multifaceted and interacting factors, and

    demonstration projects to identify effective integrated ap-
    proaches that demonstrate value, sustainability, and scalability;
- *Practice*, such as team approaches that improve outcomes, tools
  that facilitate life span approaches to the care process, reorganization of provider profiles at care entry points to improve patient
  engagement and support;
- *Education*, such as redefining core competencies, exploration of
  new care categories, and reorienting health professions training
  to emphasize prevention, well-being, and team approaches; and
- *Policy*, such as clarity on the standards of evidence that shape
  practice and payment, development of incentives that support the
  necessary developments in research, education, and practice, in
  particular those that encourage care coordination, team care, patient engagement, and an orientation to prevention and well-
  being.

A number of these suggestions are highlighted in greater detail in
later sections of this summary as reflections of the discussion but not
as consensus or recommendations, which was not the purpose of the
summit nor the intent of this summary.

SUMMIT IN BRIEF

Summit Overview and Background (Chapter 1)

Setting the stage for the summit discussions, Dr. Harvey Fineberg,
president of IOM, said that in speaking to people about integrative medicine before the summit, he felt as if he were showing them a Rorschach
blot and asking, "What do you see?" Integrative medicine, he said,
means many different things to many different people and has at least
five critical dimensions:

- *Broad definition of health:* Integrative medicine offers the possibility to fulfill the longstanding World Health Organization definition of *health* as more than the absence of disease. It should
  include physical, mental, emotional, and spiritual factors, enabling a comprehensive understanding of what makes a person
  healthy.

- *Wide range of interventions:* Integrative medicine encompasses the whole spectrum of health interventions, from prevention to treatment to rehabilitation and recovery.
- *Coordination of care:* Integrative medicine emphasizes coordination of care across an array of caregivers and institutions.
- *Patient-centered care:* Integrative medicine integrates services around and within the individual patient, which is perhaps the most fundamental and the most neglected aspect of high-quality care.
- *Variety of modalities:* Integrative medicine is open to multiple modalities of care, not just usual care, but also unconventional care that helps patients manage, maintain, and restore health.

Snyderman talked about the great difference between health and well-being and the care Americans currently experience. He acknowledged that many of the ways to improve health must be actively promoted by individuals themselves, and cannot be accomplished through the health care system. "Even the best health care system, acting alone, cannot assure good health. It needs the individual's engagement and commitment to health," he said. He described the first transformation in medical care, which occurred almost exactly 100 years ago, when advances in science resulted in the identification of microbial factors of disease and provided a new way to practice medicine. An unintended consequence of this transformation was development of the find-it-and-fix-it approach to medical treatment that focuses on identification and treatment of disease. Now, he suggested, is the time for a second transformation—one that again would be propelled by new advances in science, which for the first time are providing capabilities for quantifying health risks and the benefits of individualized therapies. This revolution could transform care into personalized, predictive, preventive, and participatory health care that would promote health and well-being.

The Vision for Integrative Health and Medicine (Chapter 2)

The panel discussion on vision underscored the notion that the current health care system is fragmented and not oriented to health promotion or disease prevention. Panel moderator, Dr. Michael Johns, for example, noted that much of today's health care system focuses on treating major, often fatal, diseases, but these efforts are not sufficient to achieve a healthy population. Bill Novelli described the large contribution that Americans' individual behavior choices make in preserving health or causing diseases. Yet, the health system is not currently geared toward supporting individuals through the long and difficult behavior change process. The health system might be more successful in eliciting behavior change if it were supported by policy changes, coordinated action across social sectors, community-based efforts, and more robust and diverse patient-education efforts, as described by Dr. Mehmet Oz. As he described his vision, Dr. Victor Sierpina noted that clinicians will need a different kind of education to work in a more integrative and community-based way.

Panelists discussed options for more integrative care efforts, including expansion of the pool of primary care providers suggested by Sierpina and use of multidisciplinary care teams. Such efforts can be greatly enhanced by electronic data systems that provide comprehensive patient-centered information to caregivers in a timely way, George Halvorson said. These systems could be the underpinning of a system for more patient-centered care. Ellen Stovall emphasized that clinicians must recognize that many of the skills patients need to actively participate in decision making about their care evaporate in the face of a serious illness, necessitating a greater need for patient-centered care that involves attention to patient preferences and integration of mind, body, and spirit.

Models of Care (Chapter 3)

In the session on models of care, speakers described various existing models of integrative care and highlighted principles that are vital to the success of future models. Speakers referred to almost a dozen different models that incorporate integrative approaches. These models have been implemented in a variety of settings and address acute care, chronic disease management, and home-based care. Throughout the session, patient-centeredness was the key theme.

In his keynote address for the session, Dr. Donald Berwick suggested that true patient-centeredness would attempt to explore patients' deep feelings about their health goals, so that care decisions would most effectively serve them and enhance prospects for successful treatments. He remarked on the notably generous spirit and common purpose reflected among summit participants, despite remarkably diverse perspectives. He underscored the importance of that sense of unity, given that the natural inclination of professional groups is to make a case for their treatment specialty, often at the expense of the patient. To avoid this fragmentation, he said, the first challenge for integrative care will be for the field to define what is being integrated, why, and then ultimately to integrate *itself*.

Drawing in part on his previous IOM committee work, Berwick proposed the following eight principles for integrative medicine:

1. Place the patient at the center.
2. Individualize care.
3. Welcome family and loved ones.
4. Maximize healing influences within care.
5. Maximize healing influences outside care.
6. Rely on sophisticated, disciplined evidence.
7. Use all relevant capacities—waste nothing.
8. Connect helping influences with each other.

Emphasizing these notions, he concluded by noting that "the sources of suffering are in separateness, and the remedy is in remembering that we are in this together."

The panel discussion was moderated by Dr. Erminia Guarneri, who opened by noting that her entire medical training was oriented to the find-it-and-fix-it mentality. Yet as she gained experience, she learned from her patients that, when it comes to cardiovascular health, the illnesses of loneliness, depression, anger, and hostility are every bit as devastating as hypertension and diabetes. She said a different model of care is needed, one that puts as much stock in the importance of social and behavioral perspectives as in lab values.

Dr. Edward Wagner agreed, noting that constructive patient–provider relationships are essential to effectively providing preventive services to individuals with established chronic illnesses, as well as those without. Wagner and others suggested that the mindset and principles of primary care may provide a sound foundation for integrative health care, but to effectively move to an integrative approach, primary care will also need to change. An important element of the transformation is to recognize that, for the 40 to 50 percent of the population suffering from chronic conditions, the distinctions between prevention and treatment begin to break down since the interventions are much the same. To foster high-quality and high-efficiency primary care, the system must include high-functioning practice teams, operate according to clear protocols, use enhanced information technology, and include structured patient involvement, said Wagner. These factors would help address the most prominent care management challenges in chronic illness care and advance toward integrative medicine.

Dr. Arnold Milstein illustrated how such approaches can be effective even in, and perhaps especially in, those settings in which the patients are sickest and poorest. He analyzed components of small medical practices (with one to two physicians, which is the type where most physicians work) and medium-sized ones (with about 60 physicians) that have effectively managed chronic diseases and controlled costs. He found that the most successful practices had certain characteristics: they worked as teams; they established close relationships with patients and provided what patients themselves perceived as personalized care; they offered some unusual services in order to address the behavioral and social elements of health care; they focused on the sickest patients in the practice and went to extraordinary effort to keep these patients out of the hospital; and they developed relationships with one or two local physicians in each specialty who practiced similarly, so that when they had to make referrals, continuity of care was maintained. He noted that each of the practices he studied could not have survived on existing fee-for-service terms and had to negotiate capitation agreements with their payers. But the result was efficient, caring experiences, delivering better outcomes at lower costs.

Dr. David Katz, Dr. Tracy Gaudet, and Dr. Mike Magee each noted that the disease-oriented approach of conventional allopathic medicine neither naturally leads to the type of clinician-patient understanding Berwick and other participants envision nor does it yield the health outcomes patients should expect. Katz noted that patients often have concerns that are in a gray zone, and the only way to effectively address them is by understanding more about the individual context of their concerns. Gaudet concurred, noting that when so much of the disease and disability among Americans is a function of personal health behavior, that the changes health professionals are asking their patients to make cannot be successful until they have deep personal significance— something she feels the current system is entirely unable to address. She said that overhauling the current health care mindset would require a physician–patient partnership, including working together to fashion a whole person medical record that embeds the key elements for planning a patient's health future, the use of teams to manage the care process, and reoriented training to make these changes possible.

In carrying this theme forward, Magee called for the notion of a home-centered health care model—one that does not have the hospital or doctor's office at the epicenter—as necessary to helping people achieve their full potential. He viewed the notion of home as both a geographic and a virtual place, and one in which complexity, connectivity, and consumerism become advantages. He pointed out the appeal of this notion by observing that "Americans abhor homelessness, yet have learned to accept healthlessness." Each of the panelists emphasized the importance of a sustained program of demonstration studies for new models, especially those that include mechanisms of payment, in moving integrative medicine forward and helping overcome the current reimbursement and cultural challenges.

Science (Chapter 4)

The session on the science base highlighted the complex interplay of biology, behavior, psychosocial factors, and how the environment shapes health and disease. The keynote address for the session was delivered by Dr. Dean Ornish, who pointed out that these interactions can produce synergistic results—for good or ill—and this complexity requires a systems approach in both health care and in health sciences research that accounts for multiple variables interacting in dynamic ways. In his presentation, Ornish described examples of various food components that seem in epidemiologic studies to either protect or promote certain disease processes. However, when studied as independent factors or administered separately, they act differently, which demonstrates that these factors do not generally act independently but in complex interdependence with other dietary components.

Ornish went on to note that various studies that examine the influence of supportive relationships and comprehensive lifestyle change suggest that not only could social and behavioral interventions change the course of a disease process, but in some circumstances could stimulate regeneration and reverse disease processes, in a dose-response fashion. Stating that nurture sometimes trumps nature, Ornish discussed some relatively new findings in genomic sciences showing the potential for lifestyle changes to affect telomere length (related to aging and longevity) and gene expression.

In the panel discussion, Dr. Nancy Adler, who reviewed the social determinants of health, picked up this theme by noting that English workers in manual occupations showed a significant decrease in telomere length relative to same-age workers in non-manual fields, indicating premature aging at the cellular level. She went on to review the powerful overall impact of income and education on health status and life expectancy, including its cross-generational influence.

A specific focus on advances in genomic sciences was provided by panelist Dr. Richard Lifton, who noted that, increasingly, new, more effective treatments that are tailored to a person's genetic profile will be available. This will greatly facilitate personalized medicine and person-centered care. Lifton noted the progress made in the 150 years since 1865 when Gregor Mendel recognized genetic factors. He offered examples of diseases such as breast cancer, Alzheimer's, hypercholesterolemia, obesity, and many others for which contributing genetic loci have been identified in the past decade. While identification of genetic variation may fragment care in the sense that it will lead to a certain level of stratification or targeting, he said it will foster an integration of approaches to the care dynamics that are important to a given individual.

Extending the notion that it is the interactions of genes with other factors (epigenetic influences) that shape health and illness, Dr. Mitchell Gaynor reported on numerous studies indicating the influence of diet and other environmental factors on the expression of genes.

The interplay of external stressors and physiologic responses was also an issue discussed by several panelists. In his introduction to the panel discussion, moderator Dr. Bruce McEwen offered an overview of how changes in levels of physiologic mediators released in the brain, such as adrenaline and cortisol, in response to stress can produce cumulative effects over time—what he termed allostatic load. McEwen noted that psychosocial factors including stress, loneliness, and depression, trigger brain-mediated responses in neural, endocrine, and immune systems, and, in time, have adverse effects on various organ systems and disease states. People with high levels of stress can be found throughout society, observed Adler, who noted that those in lower socioeconomic strata are particularly vulnerable. McEwen and Adler also described the long-term effects of stress, adverse events, and low socioeconomic status on the health of children.

Dr. Esther Sternberg noted that as the brain responds to stress, hormones are released that can interfere with the immune response and metabolic processes and damage the cardiovascular system. On the other hand, Sternberg said, something as simple as having a support group, a wide social network, or a nurturing belief system can help people manage stress and recover from illness. She said that the road to healing also is mediated by the brain. Health-promoting activities, such as meditation, yoga, tai chi, and exercise, have biologic effects on the neuroendocrine systems. When people engage in these types of activities, the vagus nerve functions as a brake on the sympathetic nervous system, thereby increasing the power of the immune system. Also, such activities prompt release of the powerful neuroendocrine system hormones—endorphins and dopamine.

Each of the panelists emphasized the potential from scientific advances and the need for studies to accelerate progress. Yet many, including Dr. Lawrence Green who was charged with reviewing research challenges, noted the complexity of studying the involved factors. In particular, this complexity presents a significant limitation to the use of randomized clinical trials, which test one variable at a time and are not designed to evaluate multifaceted preventive approaches, such as lifestyle interventions. New, more appropriate assessment methods are under development. They range from improved effectiveness trials at the community level to studies of immune system biomarkers at the molecular level, to an array of study methods being used at the National Center for Complementary and Alternative Medicine (NCCAM)—approaches that were described by the center's Director, Dr. Josephine Briggs. Briggs highlighted the four spheres of research conducted at NCCAM: basic sciences, translational research, efficacy studies, and effectiveness research, noting that approximately half of NCCAM's resources are devoted to basic research, such as studies of the neuroscience of meditation and the biology of the placebo effect.

Workforce and Education (Chapter 5)

In the summit discussion on workforce and education, speakers described the implications of advances in integrative medicine for the education and training of the nation's health professionals and researchers. They discussed strategies for changing curricula, including interdisciplinary approaches, team-based training, and expansion of core competencies in healthy living and wellness.

An often-mentioned point in this session, described by Dame Carol Black in her keynote address, is the need to expand interdisciplinary and multidisciplinary education to promote effective teamwork. Black pointed out that the only way to provide truly person-centered care is to take into account the social and economic determinants of health, which requires a very different set of provider profiles, competencies, and training. She gave, as a particular example, the importance of the relationship between work and health. Black noted that while health care providers often discuss many health behavior and environmental factors with their patients, they rarely discuss patients' employment in a meaningful way. Yet people spend more time at work than almost any other place, and it has to represent the dominant social influence on health prospects. Even more dramatic is the condition of "worklessness," which over the long term is a greater risk to health than many diseases. Overall, she emphasized, a rational approach to health care requires a team approach, in order to address both the growing complexity in diagnosis and treatment interventions and the similarly complex social and behavioral factors affecting health.

Dr. Elizabeth Goldblatt echoed this theme, noting that people and patients desire collaboration among their health care providers, which presumes innovative multidisciplinary educational experiences, training, and guidelines for all licensed health professionals. Yet, health practitioners typically are educated and trained in professional silos, hindering their ability to quickly transition and adapt to a team environment. Interprofessional education should begin early, particularly for physicians, to reinforce shared values and overcome the culture that rewards individual accomplishment, said Dr. Adam Perlman, who detailed the related approaches, barriers, and opportunities.

To inform the change process, demonstration projects were noted as useful in developing more effective educational models for integrative health practitioners. Dr. Mary Jo Kreitzer, who sees the necessity for disruptive innovation in both health professions education and health care delivery, suggested that community health centers be incorporated into interdisciplinary education experiences. Another approach would involve training nonphysicians to be primary care providers. Dr. Richard Cooper viewed this prospect as inevitable and critical, because of the looming shortage of primary care physicians. Expanded primary care capacity might be achieved by developing new competencies for nurse practitioners and others. Dr. Victoria Maizes suggested training programs built around core competencies in integrative health. Maizes discussed several related approaches but noted that much work is to be done in forging and getting agreement on a competency-based curriculum of the sort needed.

Underscoring the need for a new look at competencies and curriculum was the fact that, regardless of professional and specialty mix, health care practitioners today are not able to overcome some of the most important factors in health and disease, including the socioeconomic factors raised by Black. In many respects, Cooper said, poverty constitutes the greatest of all the challenges facing the health care system. In fact, approximately 17 percent of all Americans and 21 percent of their children live in poverty, ranking the United States with the third highest rates of poverty overall and fourth highest rates of poverty for children among OECD[2] nations (OECD, 2009).

Sir Cyril Chantler addressed the question of legal and regulatory implications inherent in a move toward integrative medicine. Chantler noted the need to ensure an adequate evidence base as a precondition for the integrative practice and its oversight. But he also noted the need for standards appropriately tailored to the individual issue at hand, with patient safety the top priority. However, evaluation needs to go beyond this to address questions of benefit and cost-effectiveness. One of the challenges is to ensure that the consideration of benefit includes individual patient values. In the matter of credentialing, Chantler noted that standards for professional competence should be clear and consistent, that outcomes should be carefully recorded and audited, and that teamwork capacity should be an essential element.

In a comment that reflected the overall spirit of the discussion and the need for action, Chantler acknowledged the importance of the axiom *primum non nocere,* "first do no harm," but also added another, *deinde adjuvare,* "next do some good."

Economics and Policy (Chapter 6)

The keynote address for the session on economic and policy issues was delivered by Senator Tom Harkin who shared his optimism about meaningful health reform by referring to President Obama's recent remarks before a joint session of Congress, in which he predicted that Congress would pass a comprehensive health reform measure in 2009 and that the centerpiece of the reform would be a new emphasis on prevention and wellness. Harkin noted that, unlike previous occasions, public sentiment is now clearly that the health care system is substantially dysfunctional and in need of dramatic change. He called for a system that emphasizes care coordination and continuity, patient-centeredness, holis-

---

[2]Organisation for Economic and Co-operation and Development.

tic approaches, and wellness. Such an integrative approach, he said, would take advantage of the very best scientifically based practices, whether conventional or alternative. It would focus on the twin goals of improving outcomes and reducing costs.

In the following panel discussion, Dr. Kenneth Thorpe reiterated that changes outside the health system (e.g., environmental and food policy) can have a profound effect on health, and that there is an opportunity for reforms in these areas to be included in an administration-wide discussion of health reform. For every dollar spent on medical costs for treating chronic diseases, many of which are preventable, he suggested, another $4 is lost through decreased productivity. He acknowledged the difficulty that small physician practices have in providing services such as care coordination, primary prevention, and community outreach, and supported development of community health teams that would include nurse practitioners, social workers, and behavioral health workers to collaborate with these practices to make these services available.

Dr. Janet Kahn also suggested greater coordination of health-promoting activities across government agencies, including agencies outside of the Department of Health and Human Services, as part of the reform process. In discussing the political and policy realities, panelists cautioned that health reform, especially reform emphasizing integrative concepts, is far from a certainty. As a tactical matter, Tom Donohue warned against pointing fingers at other sectors and advised that advocates unite around commonly held values.

Dr. Reed Tuckson emphasized that health insurance companies have agendas and missions that are well aligned with the summit's goals, and noted that his own company, UnitedHealth Group, views itself as "a health and well-being company." His emphasis was on the need for evidence on workable models that could be used to support changes in financing. When thinking about integrative medicine, he asked for clarity in how different members of the comprehensive care team are to be trained, credentialed, evaluated, coordinated, coded, and reimbursed, and how redundancy would be minimized and efficiency improved.

Donohue said that businesses today are supportive of health system change. For insurers and the business community alike, the dominant concern is rising health care costs. Donohue and William George both viewed the business community as strong participants in reforming the health system, not only because of their traditional insurance role, but also because of their successes with employee wellness programs. George noted that the goal for employers that emphasize wellness is not achieving the lowest cost for employee health benefits; it is to have 100 percent of employees fully present on the job every day—in other words, improved productivity. The starting point for that productivity is a corporate culture where health is honored and enjoyed.

Examples of the ways successful programs have not only improved employee health but also demonstrated return on investment to employers were described by Dr. Kenneth Pelletier. He reported on research that identified 153 clinical and cost outcome studies of worksite integrative health approaches, all of which demonstrated net benefits with respect to short- and long-term disability, absenteeism, personnel retention, presenteeism, and performance. Pelletier noted that the studies he reviewed reflected returns on investment ranging from 3.5 to 4.9:1. He suggested approaches that might be used to further evaluate the potential economic returns from integrative programs.

Concluding Comments (Chapter 7)

The final session of the summit was devoted to an open review of key points of the summit discussions, including a panel conversation among the moderators of the five previous summit sessions, followed by closing comments from Fineberg and Snyderman. In the panel discussion, participants noted the clear emphasis throughout the summit on reorientation of care to perspectives that emphasized prevention, were person centered and life span long, accommodated multidisciplinary team engagement, and tended to the social, home, and relationship environments so important in influencing individual and population health.

Participants also identified considerations of particular importance moving forward. Johns, for example, noted that a challenge was to avoid piling an entirely new set of practitioner tools onto existing practice patterns. Rather, in integrative *health* an entirely new orientation is needed, including the involvement of an "optimizer"—human and/or electronic—devoted to ensuring that the right intervention is provided at the right time and the most appropriate place. Guarneri commented that the practitioner's toolbox has to be equipped with much more than drugs and devices. Instead, it needs to be designed as a community kit for use in a care model drawing on multidisciplinary teams. However, considerable work would need to be done to bring credentialing and financial incentives into alignment with the vision.

In addressing the issue of involving multiple disciplines, McEwen remarked on the impressive promise of advancing science, if it can break free from the tendency toward specialization and reductionism, but he cautioned that engaging truly interdisciplinary perspectives and activities is very challenging. The signals must be strong from field leaders, in training programs, and from funding sources. Goldblatt again stated the importance of beginning very early in the professional training process with priorities, emphases, and skills directed to wellness and to under-standing the range of factors in play for the whole patient, not just the physiologic correlates of the presenting symptom. She noted that if peo-ple are educated in silos, they will practice in silos, and that style of prac-tice in increasingly untenable.

Tunis reminded participants that the United States is faced with a once-in-a-generation opportunity for major political and social change on behalf of better health care. He noted that the economic challenges may in fact be working to counter a culture of greed and shift to greater reso-nance with the values of integrative medicine—internal reflection, con-nectedness, and community support. He also cautioned that sustaining the "shared sympathy" of the discussions would be a challenge, but it was very important, given the natural inclination in resource-related dis-cussions to point fingers and place blame across sectors. Finally, he pre-dicted that integrative medicine may turn out to be the most successful approach to reforming the nation's health system.

In their concluding remarks, Snyderman, chair of the summit plan-ning committee, and Fineberg, president of the IOM, both thanked all of the participants for their time, their active engagement, and their energy and enthusiasm throughout the summit. Snyderman and Fineberg said the event was far bigger and far more important than the organizers could have anticipated when they began the initiative more than a year earlier.

Returning to the Rorschach blot that Fineberg discussed in his open-ing remarks, Snyderman reiterated that everyone had arrived at the meet-ing with some image of integrative medicine. Those images were probably different in virtually every mind, and while the summit had not led to a precise and universally accepted view of integrative health care—nor was that the intention—it had clearly led to much greater un-derstanding, to identification of common elements, and to appreciation that at its center is an individual with unique requirements for maintain-ing health, preventing disease, and health care services. Snyderman said that the unique individual is each of us over the course of our lifetimes; it is our friends and family members; and it is every one of the nation's children, with their different socioeconomic backgrounds and opportunities, their different racial and ethnic identities, their different family dynamics, and their different futures.

Snyderman also noted that Fineberg was wise to ask people, near the end of the plenary, what they had learned, what for them was different. He concluded by saying that "to some degree all of our minds have been changed, unalterably. We are different people, capable of taking different actions. Much of what comes out of the summit will depend on the spontaneous actions and the creativity of every person in the audience. We all can play a role in keeping this movement going forward."

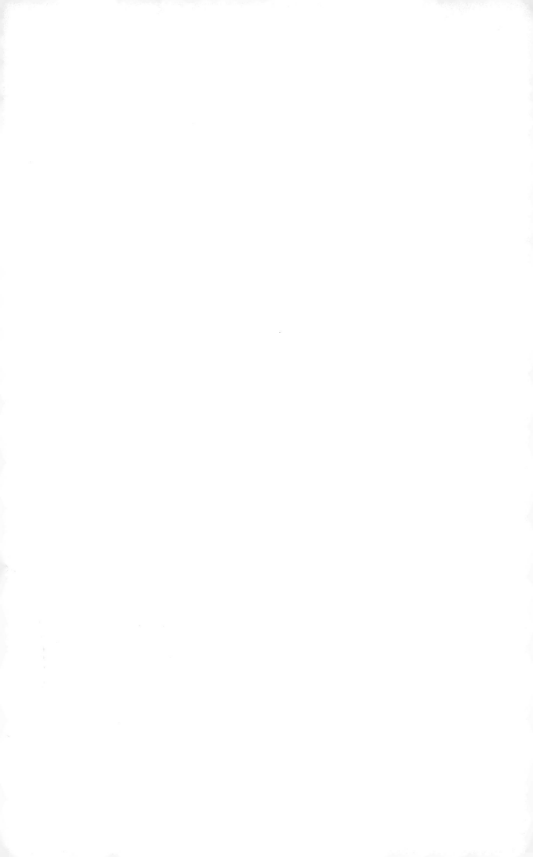

1

Summit Overview and Background

INTRODUCTION

The last century witnessed dramatic changes in the practice of health care, and coming decades promise advances that were not imaginable even in the relatively recent past. Science and technology continue to offer new insights into disease pathways and treatments, as well as mechanisms of protecting health and preventing disease. Genomics and proteomics are bringing personalized risk assessment, prevention, and treatment options within reach; health information technology is expediting the collection and analysis of large amounts of data that can lead to improved care; and many disciplines are contributing to a broadening understanding of the complex interplay among biology, environment, behavior, and socioeconomic factors that shape health and wellness.

Although medical advances have saved and improved the lives of millions, much of medicine and health care have primarily focused on addressing immediate events of disease and injury, generally neglecting underlying socioeconomic factors, including employment, education, and income, and behavioral risk factors. These factors, and others, impact health status, accentuate disparities, and can lead to costly, preventable diseases (IOM, 2001b). Furthermore, the disease-driven approach to medicine and health care has resulted in a fragmented, specialized health system in which care is typically reactive and episodic, as well as often inefficient and impersonal (IOM, 2007b; Snyderman and Williams, 2003).

In health terms, the consequences of this fragmentation can be serious. Chronic conditions now represent the major challenge to the U.S. health care system. Five chronic conditions—diabetes, heart disease, asthma, high blood pressure, and depression—account for more than half of all U.S. health expenditures (Druss et al., 2001). Among Medicare recipients, 20 percent live with five or more chronic conditions and their care accounts for two-thirds of all Medicare expenditures (Anderson, 2005). Many of these conditions are preventable, but only about 55 percent of the most recommended clinical preventive services are actually delivered (McGlynn et al., 2003).

Care coordination that emphasizes wellness and prevention, a hallmark of integrative medicine, is a major and growing need for people both with and without chronic diseases. Those with chronic diseases rarely receive the full support they need to achieve maximum benefit. A patient's course of care may require contact with clinicians and caregivers and may require many transitions, for example from hospital to home care. However, these transitions often are poorly handled, leading to adverse events that result in rehospitalizations 20 percent of the time (Forster et al., 2003). The IOM report *To Err is Human* concluded that half of all adverse events are caused by preventable medical errors. Indeed, it estimated that medical errors are responsible for some 44,000 to 98,000 deaths per year, ranking errors among the nation's leading causes of death (IOM, 1999).

Disconnected and uncoordinated care amplifies the economic burden of the health care system. The costs of U.S. health care are driven in large part by the inefficiencies, redundancies, and excesses of the current fragmented system and are considered by many economists and policy makers to be unsustainable, either for individuals or for the nation. In 2009, nearly $2.5 trillion will be spent in the United States in a health care system that is underperforming on many dimensions. The current trend will drive expenditures to $4.3 trillion by 2017 (Keehan et al., 2008) unless changes are made. Despite per capita expenditures that are at least twice as high as the average for other Western nations, the United States ranks far down the global list in the health of its citizens (Schoen et al., 2006). Estimates by various experts suggest that one-third to one-half of U.S. health expenditures do little to improve health (U.S. Congress, 2004; U.S. Congress, 2006).

Combined, economic challenges and dissatisfaction with the current system drive interest in health reforms that would offer lower-cost, more effective, holistic, evidence-based approaches. This interest is growing concurrent with, and fueled by, growth in the science base about the relationships among health, the pace of healing, and more intangible elements of the caring process, including empowerment of patients to play a central role in their care. Evidence is accumulating about the variety of factors that have important effects on health care outcomes: the interaction between an individual's social, economic, psychological, and physical environments, and his or her biological susceptibility to illness and responsiveness to treatment; the nature of the care *process*, as well as its *content*; and the often greater health benefit to be had from certain "lower tech" interventions, rather than more costly approaches.

In addition, the interest in unconventional approaches to prevention and treatment has grown. In 2007, nearly two of every five Americans over the age of 18 reported use of therapies such as yoga, massage, meditation, and natural products and supplements (Barnes et al., 2008). In total, such approaches accounted for $34 billion in out-of-pocket expenditures in 2007 (Nahin et al., 2009). And, more than half of all Americans over the age of 18 report regular use of dietary supplements, supporting a $23 billion industry (National Institutes of Health, 2006). Some of these practices are based on the experience of cultures over time, some are based on evolving scientific theories, and some are based on little more than belief. Each compels an assessment of what is lacking in conventional health care that causes so many people to turn elsewhere for help. Stakeholders must determine which models and approaches to health care, conventional or otherwise, might best integrate the science, caring, efficiency, and results that patients desire and that improve optimal health and well-being throughout the life span.

This is the background to the IOM's Summit on Integrative Medicine and the Health of the Public. Integrative medicine may be described as orienting the health care process to create a seamless engagement by patients and caregivers of the full range of physical, psychological, social, preventive, and therapeutic factors known to be effective and necessary for the achievement of optimal health throughout the life span. The aim of the meeting was to explore opportunities, challenges, and models for a more integrative approach to health and medicine. This approach could shift the focus of the health care system toward efficient, evidence-based practice, prevention, wellness, and patient-centered care, creating a more personalized, predictive, and participatory health care experience.

THE SUMMIT ON INTEGRATIVE MEDICINE
AND THE HEALTH OF THE PUBLIC

The IOM Summit on Integrative Medicine and the Health of the Public was sponsored by the Bravewell Collaborative and was planned by a 14-member planning committee, chaired by Dr. Ralph Snyderman.[1] The summit was designed to consider integrative content to a number of initiatives for transforming the health care system, including

- patient-centered care;
- personalized, predictive, preventive, participatory medicine;
- mind–body relationships;
- the scientific basis of integrative medicine;
- health care financing reform;
- shared decision making;
- value-driven health care; and
- and team-based care processes.

The agenda was divided into five half-day sessions, each with a keynote speaker, a panel of expert presenters, and audience discussion. The plenary sessions covered overarching visions for integrative medicine, models of care, workforce and education needs, and economic and policy implications.

The planning committee worked to ensure sufficient time for discussion and active audience engagement, believing that the success of the summit would be measured by the quality of the presentations as well as the level of participant engagement. Panelists' formal presentations were limited to 8 minutes, but each panel included ample time for further discussion among the panelists and with the audience. Eight lunch sessions served as open discussion forums for all summit participants and involved no structured presentations. Each lunch discussion was hosted by two or three discussion leaders, many of whom were summit panelists; the topics of discussion ranged from the health care reform agenda to evaluating the evidence base to enhancing wellness to mind–body and societal connections. A complete list of discussion topics and leaders is in Appendix C.

---

[1]The role of the planning committee was limited to planning and preparation of the summit. This document was prepared by rapporteurs as a factual summary of what was presented and discussed at the summit.

To further expand on the summit discussion and to begin identifying challenges and opportunities for the future of integrative medicine, the planning committee assembled five priority assessment groups. These groups' topics reflected the five summit panels: health reform, models, science, workforce and education, and economic incentives. Assessment groups were asked to address the following questions:

- What are the three most important priorities in addressing this topic?
- Who are the key actors for implementation and their roles?
- What might be the achievable 3-year and 10-year goals?
- What are the next steps?

The assessment groups met during the lunch sessions to respond to these questions. Each group had a moderator, a rapporteur, and approximately 10 expert members holding a variety of views on the topic at hand. A list of priority assessment group participants is in Appendix C. Chapters 2 through 6 of this summary include the priority assessment group reports, which are based on the rapporteurs' presentations to the plenary sessions and the ensuing discussion of summit participants. These reports reflect the priorities discussed and presented by the assessment group, not recommendations from the summit.

WELCOME AND CHARGE TO SUMMIT PARTICIPANTS
Harvey V. Fineberg, Institute of Medicine

Summit participants were welcomed by Dr. Harvey Fineberg, president of the IOM, who noted that the summit constituted the largest, most diverse, and quite possibly the most enthusiastic audience ever assembled by the IOM. He expressed appreciation to the Bravewell Collaborative for its support in making the summit possible.

In speaking to people about integrative medicine before the summit, Fineberg said he felt as if he were showing them a Rorschach blot and asking, "What do you see?" Integrative medicine, he said, means many different things to many different people and has at least five critical dimensions:

1. *Broad definition of health:* Integrative medicine offers the possibility to fulfill the longstanding World Health Organization defi-

nition of *health* as more than the absence of disease. It embraces
the physical, mental, emotional, and spiritual factors, enabling a
comprehensive understanding of what makes a person healthy.

2. *Wide range of interventions:* Integrative medicine encompasses a
full spectrum of health interventions and all factors that contribute to health. It includes approaches to prevention, to treatment,
to rehabilitation, and to recovery.

3. *Coordination of care:* Integrative medicine emphasizes coordination of care across an array of caregivers and institutions.

4. *Patient-centered care:* Integrative medicine integrates services
around and within the individual patient, putting patients and
their needs at the center. Patient-centered care is perhaps the
most fundamental aspect of the six dimensions of high-quality
care that were defined by *Crossing the Quality Chasm: A New
Health System for the 21st Century* (IOM, 2001a).

5. *Variety of modalities:* Integrative medicine is open to multiple
modalities of care, not just "usual care," but also unconventional
care that helps patients manage, maintain, and restore health.

Fineberg emphasized that these five dimensions must be supported
by a strong foundation of sound evidence. Many scientists and traditionally trained allopathic physicians are skeptical of the benefits of integrative medicine. Fineberg noted that he, too, is skeptical, but that he is also
skeptical of claims about what works in conventional medicine. He suggested that the same standard of evidence must be applied to any proposed idea about what will and will not work in health care, including
conventional care.

Throughout the history of public health and medicine, Fineberg
noted that there are examples of interventions that were known to be effective at the time, despite a lack of understanding of the mechanisms by
which the interventions operated. In 19th-century Europe, when many
people believed that disease was spread by *miasmas*, early sanitarians
struggled to separate sewage and drinking water. Only later was the germ
theory established, leading to the identification of the biological cause of
these diseases. "They were right for the wrong reason," Fineberg said of
the sanitarians, adding that "Sometimes it is better to be right for the
wrong reason than to be wrong for the right reason."

Some commonly used treatments have evolved from traditional
herbal remedies whose mechanisms were likewise unknown in earlier
times. For example, the earliest effective treatment of malaria, quinine,

was derived from the bark of the Amazon's cinchona tree. Contemporary malaria treatment is based on artemisinin, an ingredient derived from Chinese herbal medicine. The dividing line for acceptance of a therapeutic method, therefore, is not about its origin or even the theory behind it; the dividing line must be the evidence, said Fineberg.

What unites the five dimensions of integrative medicine and the necessary reliance on evidence is a philosophy of health and health care. This philosophy embraces the patient at the center; it talks about prevention, as well as treatment; it integrates across institutions and caregivers; it is open to a variety of modalities, so long as they work; and it defines integrative medicine.

KEYNOTE ON INTEGRATING HEALTH AND HEALTH CARE
Ralph Snyderman, Duke University

> *There is nothing more difficult to plan, more doubtful of success, nor more dangerous to manage than the creation of a new system. The initiator has the enmity of all who profit from the old institution and merely the lukewarm defenders in those who would gain the new ones.*
> *—Machiavelli*

Health is fundamental to virtually everything that people do and is perhaps one's most important resource. As the World Health Organization has long avowed, health is more than absence of disease. Good health, Dr. Ralph Snyderman suggested, is a source of vigor, robustness, and well-being, and it generates the will and capacity to do things. Achieving good health is not a function of the health care system alone; to a large extent, individuals have control over the state of their own health. Many diseases can be prevented and, if they develop, be mitigated by actions people take on their own as well as through therapeutic and wellness plans in collaboration with and aided by their health care providers. Rational transformation of the current disconnected approach to health care, said Snyderman, will require a seamless integration of resources to empower individuals to improve their health, while providing the resources needed to prevent and treat disease.

Health vs. Health Care

As health care has grown to a $2.5 trillion a year industry in the United States, this rapid expansion has led to serious economic turmoil, said Snyderman. This turmoil affects all Americans, including the 47 million who do not have health insurance; employers, who cannot afford to offer insurance or whose businesses strain from insurance costs; providers, who see their own costs rising uncontrollably; and payers, especially government payers, with Medicare and Medicaid consuming larger and larger shares of public resources. Rising unemployment rates are likely to cause the number of uninsured and underinsured to grow substantially, further distorting the health care system, noted Snyderman.

If these large national expenditures produced a well-operating health care system and good health outcomes for patients, the expenditures might be considered worthwhile, despite the high cost. However, U.S. health statistics, the system's poor safety record, and patient dissatisfaction indicate overall dysfunction and a lack of value, said Snyderman. Numerous frequently recognized problems in the U.S. health system directly hinder a focus on "health." The current system, he said, is oriented toward treating disease events in an uncoordinated fashion, rather than toward prevention or coherent disease management. In addition, care is neither personalized nor standardized; it lacks coordination across providers and poses difficulties navigating among them; it does not engage patients in decision making; and, in many instances, it has proved unsafe.

Snyderman said that the health system *should*, first of all, focus on promoting and enhancing health and well-being, on identifying susceptibilities, and on reducing risks for chronic disease. When health problems arise, the system should intervene early, provide the best available care for acute events, deal effectively and holistically with chronic conditions, and ensure compassionate support at the end of life. The current health care system is now capable of this full range of services, he said, but it does few of them in a coordinated manner.

Health and the Individual

Fundamentally, integrative medicine brings individuals to the center of their own care over the course of their life. Health risks and strengths are unique to each person. Even though, as humans, we have 99 percent of our genes in common, we differ in terms of our susceptibility to chronic diseases, in our exposure to environmental conditions, and in our access to and use of health-related services. However, Snyderman noted that the current U.S. system is ill equipped to provide personalized care that addresses each person's unique circumstances, characteristics, and needs. The health care system has focused on developing new diagnostic and treatment capabilities—and the system has developed many remarkable ones. But, he says, little thought is given to applying these capabilities to a patient's unique needs over a lifetime and delivering them effectively and systematically for each individual.

Even the best health care system, acting alone, cannot assure good health. Snyderman noted that many dimensions of a person's life must also be considered and seamlessly engaged. These dimensions include the full range of factors that affect optimal health over a lifetime—physical, cognitive, psychological, social, and spiritual. For the health system to develop the services that will more effectively promote health and well-being, Snyderman said that it will need to take this broader range of factors into account, through a tighter integration of systems, more comprehensive therapeutic approaches, and development of a health care workforce with more diverse skills.

Bringing individuals into the center of their own care will require health practitioners to work with patients to create their own strategic personal health plans based on their personal health needs. Snyderman observed that while Americans plan for retirement or vacation, few develop plans for their most valuable resource—their health. Effective personal health planning requires individuals to better understand their role in protecting health and to assume more responsibility for it. It also requires that they work with their health providers to assess the factors—both internal (personal strengths and health risks) and external (what the health system and their social setting can provide)—affecting their health potential, noted Snyderman.

A New Transformation

Current shortcomings in the U.S. health system call for a significant transformation, said Snyderman. The first transformation in U.S. medicine occurred in the early 1900s and was the culmination of many powerful scientific discoveries that emerged decades earlier. Development of the germ theory substantiated the role of microbial agents in the development of disease; discoveries in chemistry helped scientists go from concoctions of tree bark to specific chemical treatments; understanding of physiology and pathology increased markedly and better explained disease development and classification; and advances in physics enabled imaging and radiology. These remarkable scientific leaps, however, inadvertently fostered the reductionist idea that for every complex disease there is a single cause, and doctors should find it and fix it, said Snyderman. Thus, health care became set on the path to where we are today, with all the benefits and unforeseen consequences.

In business, the find-it-and-fix-it approach is called the *root cause analysis* of failure. In health care, these failures are events of disease. Snyderman noted that no business would plan or run its operations exclusively based on a successive series of failures. Successful businesses develop strategic plans to achieve success, improve performance, and avoid failures. Health care, likewise, should be based on strategic, systemic, and systematic plans to improve health and prevent as many failures as possible. To a great degree, he said, health care providers are increasingly capable of doing this.

While the focus on finding and fixing was vital to understanding disease and developing treatments in those early years, this focus is now too narrow and insufficient to work with complex chronic diseases. A second transformation in medicine, to deal with the complexity and dynamic nature of chronic diseases, is possible and overdue, noted Snyderman. This transformation, again, would be propelled by and greatly dependent on the power of science. Genomics, proteomics, metabolomics, and systems biology now lead the way in the biological sciences. The information sciences provide the ability to accumulate and analyze mass amounts of information. Microprocessing and nanoprocessing offer new analytic capabilities that were impossible even a decade ago. These advances in science and technology can allow clinicians to anticipate negative health events before they occur, personalize prevention and treatment, identify individuals highly susceptible to specific chronic diseases, and develop

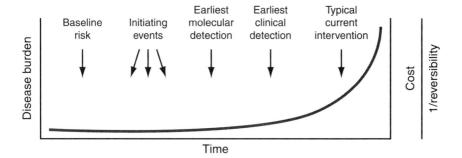

FIGURE 1-1 The inflection curve demonstrating the dynamic nature of chronic disease.
NOTES: The x-axis is time, so interventions further to the right occur later in the progress of a disease, and the y-axis represents the disease burden, cost of care, and reversibility. In this diagram, interventions that appear closer to the top cost more and are less likely to reverse disease progress. At present, interventions typically occur late along the x-axis, where the curve starts to pitch upward. These late interventions generate the high costs and low reversibility indicative of advancing chronic disease.

BOX 1-1
The Inflection Curve Case Study

Snyderman further illustrated the inflection curve concept by describing the case of a hypothetical, but all too typical, 55-year-old man who walks into an emergency room with crushing chest pain. He is given appropriate, but costly, treatment—thrombolytic therapy, stenting, bypass surgery, or medical therapy—and survives his heart attack. He may well go on to develop congestive heart failure in the following years. While this potentially catastrophic event occurred at age 55, he probably had fatty streaks in his aorta at age 25 and started developing atherosclerosis soon afterward. He may even have been born with a susceptibility to coronary artery disease; perhaps his parents died early due to the same condition. Although the health care system did not intervene until after a serious event, the opportunity to help him started far earlier along the inflection curve—when care would have been much less costly and more effective.

If our patient's heart attack, despite therapy, leads to significant heart damage, he may enter a period of seriously declining health as a consequence of congestive heart failure. If so, the system still should be able to intervene in ways that benefit him more and cost less than high-tech rescue efforts that merely focus on disease events rather than coherent disease management. In short, the health system could and should anticipate the full spectrum of this man's needs, across the life span: prevention, early intervention, more coherent and compassionate disease management, and excellent end-of-life care.

plans to mitigate them. In short, health care today can build on and improve what was developed a century ago, in order to become a personalized, predictive, and preventive care system that promotes health and well-being, as is illustrated in Figure 1-1 and Box 1-1.

Next Steps

Solutions to the current health system problems described will not be entirely high-tech. Indeed, Snyderman suggested that much of what is needed are low-tech solutions: efforts to improve individuals' knowledge about their health and increase their understanding of their role in preserving and enhancing it, and strengthening and coordinating support systems. Central to this approach is personalized health planning and the support needed to carry out individualized plans.

Snyderman said that the process could begin with a shift in the usual patient–physician encounter, from the emphasis on find it and fix it to strategic health planning that integrates an assessment of current health status, risk for various diseases, tracking, and development of wellness plans, and, when needed, therapeutic plans. In general, Snyderman said, health care providers would serve as mentors, help promote changes in lifestyle, and provide specific needed clinical services—all aided by a patient navigator or health coach. Depending on circumstances, the coach may be the primary care provider, another health expert, or even an automated or online interactive service.

While the nation's health system must continue to rest on a sound foundation of scientific evidence and must retain the benefits of new scientific knowledge and technological innovation, science and technology *alone* can resolve only a small fraction of the problems that patients experience and clinicians see daily, he said. The patient–provider encounter must also be characterized by care, compassion, understanding, and humility, in order to support the full range of patients' health and wellness needs. In part, Snyderman noted, humility requires being open to evidence from a variety of sources, weighing it objectively, and using it where circumstances warrant.

Darwin did not say that the strongest members of a species survive, as commonly believed, but that the survivors are *the ones most responsive to change.* Change in a system that accounts for almost 20 percent of the U.S. economy and affects every person in the country, may seem impossible at times, said Snyderman, and many forces will try to block the kind of transformation described. Nevertheless, in the current economic and political climate, health care reform seems possible, and perhaps even inevitable. "Either it will happen slowly, or it will happen more quickly," Snyderman said. "What we want is to see that it happens quickly and rationally."

2

The Vision for Integrative Health and Medicine

An ounce of prevention is worth a pound of cure.
—Benjamin Franklin

Against the backdrop of Ralph Snyderman's opening description of his vision for a more integrated health care system, a panel of national health care leaders offered their visions of the key dimensions of integrative medicine. Moderated by Michael Johns, the panelists emphasized the notion that the current health care system is fragmented, short sighted, and not oriented to health promotion or disease prevention, and that a shift in the focus of the system will be necessary for a healthy population. Bill Novelli, for example, described the large contribution that Americans' individual behavior choices make in preserving health or causing diseases. Yet, the health system is not currently geared toward supporting individuals through the long and difficult behavior change process. The health system might be more successful in eliciting behavior change if it were supported by policy changes, coordinated action across social sectors, community-based efforts, and more robust and diverse patient-education efforts, as described by Dr. Mehmet Oz. Dr. Victor Sierpina also noted that clinicians will need a different kind of education to work in a more integrative and community-based way.

Panelists discussed options for more integrative care efforts, including multidisciplinary care teams. Such efforts can be greatly enhanced by electronic data systems that provide comprehensive patient-centered information to caregivers in a timely way, George Halvorson said. These systems could be the underpinning of a system for more patient-centered care. Ellen Stovall emphasized that clinicians must recognize that many of the skills patients need to actively participate in decision making about their care evaporate in the face of a serious illness, necessitating a greater measure of commitment by their clinicians and caregivers.

PANEL ON THE VISION FOR INTEGRATIVE MEDICINE

Panel Introduction
Michael M. E. Johns, Emory University

Dr. Johns began the vision panel with a brief review of life expectancy and causes of death. Each year, heart disease causes one death out of every five, and cancer, one out of every seven. While death is a certainty for everyone, life expectancy and cause of death vary greatly due to individual risk and exposure. Not surprisingly, much of today's health care system focuses on treating the major, often fatal, diseases. However, these efforts are not sufficient to achieve a healthy population, said Johns.

What the health system should seek to accomplish is demonstrated by the "square wave life curve" (Figure 2-1). This curve is the ideal lifespan experience—from birth, through a long, healthy life, and then a rapid decline and death at age 120 (in this illustration). The longest confirmed life span in history was that of Jeanne Calment, of Arles, France, who died at age 122. She lived a remarkably healthy and active life for

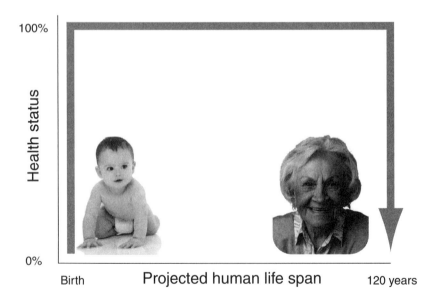

FIGURE 2-1 The square wave life curve.

nearly that entire period; in a sense, she lived the square life curve. To achieve this ideal, the health system would have to concentrate more on wellness, health, prevention, and just plain living, bringing these factors into balance with the attention currently paid to diagnosing and treating disease. Johns noted that this concept of lifelong health could transform health care and would serve humanity well.

Johns encouraged a reconsideration of some of the common terms used to describe our current health care system, in order to better align the terms with the envisioned health care system of the future. He noted that the term *medical*, as in *medical care*, often excludes the many other health-related professions. To improve the nomenclature, he would replace *evidence-based medicine* with *evidence-based health care*, *medical home* with *health home*, and *integrative medicine* with *integrative health and health care*.

Health Promotion and Disease Prevention
William D. Novelli, AARP

Successful health care reform and implementation of an integrative health model will require an increased emphasis on health promotion and disease prevention. Research by the National Business Group on Health indicates that, in 2000, almost 47 percent of U.S. deaths were caused by modifiable health behavior, including tobacco use, poor diet, and physical inactivity (National Business Group on Health, 2007). These types of behavior are strong risk factors in all three leading causes of death: heart disease, cancer, and stroke. A coherent set of national health goals and strategies and an effective program for health promotion and disease prevention could provide one of the biggest returns on investment this nation could ever make, said Novelli.

Substantial changes in health behavior would require a synergistic combination of social marketing and public policy strategies that reach beyond the clinical setting. Broad changes would be required in the environments in which people actually work, live, and play. These places include supermarkets, convenience stores, classrooms, playgrounds, factories, and especially couches, where people are influenced by a barrage of media messages from television, video games, movies, computers, cell phones, and personal digital assistants (PDAs). These places are where behavior is set, where habits are formed, and where peer and other influences take place; they are also where healthy behavior must become normative.

To counter these influences, marketing programs and policy changes can encourage people to take the steps that will lead to good health. An IOM report, *Ending the Tobacco Problem: A Blueprint for the Nation* (2007a), for example, recommended combined marketing and policy strategies to reduce the use of tobacco. The policy changes included federal regulation of manufacturing, marketing, and sales of tobacco products; tax increases; and local interventions. The social marketing strategies recommended would combine with public policy and medical strategies to create more effective smoking cessation programs that go beyond the typical medical model.

Although much of the discussion around prevention focuses on whether it adds to or reduces health care costs, the point of prevention is to maximize Americans' health potential. It will take national leadership to refocus the health system on the problems and costs of preventable conditions. While government programs are important, the nation will also need true public-private partnerships. These partnerships must include not just traditional health and medical entities but other relevant stakeholders—from educators, policy makers, insurance companies, drug manufacturers, and the news media to corporations, including the fast food and processed food industries, and those who influence our agricultural subsidies.

Novelli said that the nation has been shortsighted in not supporting

- wider use of clinical preventive services (screenings, immunizations, guidance on preventive actions);
- public, patient, and physician education programs on important risk factors such as hypertension; and
- successful public campaigns such as youth tobacco control initiatives.

Novelli said that the government also must redress the fragmentation of its current prevention efforts, which involve numerous federal and state agencies and produce little coherence, no synergy, and no "home-run power." A more coherent approach across agencies and clearer prevention targets might help solve one of the field's biggest challenges: We often know what to do, but we are not very good at getting people to do it.

Integrative Infrastructure and Systems
George Halvorson, Kaiser Permanente

According to George Halvorson, one of the keys to advancing integrative health will be to develop a toolkit of relevant systems, infrastructure, and support. Integrative health care not only requires patient-centered services, but also patient-centered data systems and information, as shown in Figure 2-2. By putting the patient at the center of health care transactions, health care providers can begin to overcome the silos within both specialty-based medical care and the various disciplines involved in alternative care. In a patient-centered data system, every patient is a data point from which much can be learned.

Ideally, electronic data systems and health records would make patient information available to every relevant caregiver in real time, which encourages and enables service integration, said Halvorson. The American Recovery and Reinvestment Act of 2009 included support for electronic patient records and electronic support for care, which could move this effort forward. However, the emphasis must be on information systems that link with one another and share data across geography and providers. New systems must not be allowed to simply replicate the problems inherent in the old, isolated paper medical records.

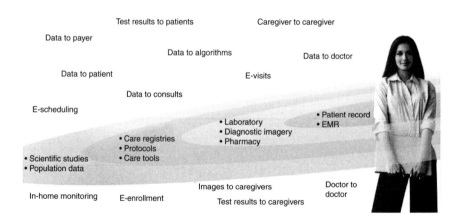

FIGURE 2-2 Care that revolves around you.
NOTES: Comprehensive data connections to every part of the system: all the info, about all of the patients, all of the time.

The infrastructure for truly integrated care will also require health professionals to work more effectively in teams. These teams can include a variety of caregivers—nurses, physicians, primary care providers, specialists, pharmacists, and alternative practitioners. These teams should be capable of effectively reacting to medical incidents, but also capable of identifying and communicating the broad set of actions required for patients to improve their health. This, in part, depends on applying data from patients' comprehensive electronic health records (EHRs) to assess risks, design behavior change options, and optimize opportunities for better health.

At Kaiser Permanente, for example, EHRs incorporate algorithms that analyze patients' data to create individualized support tools for care. The tools are used by teams of caregivers across the health care setting as they actively work with and advise individual patients. Personalized information is used in selecting treatments but also may be used in suggesting behavior changes, best weight and activity levels, and other health promotion opportunities. In its Colorado region, using intensified team care that is guided by patients' own data, Kaiser has experienced a 72 percent reduction in deaths from heart disease.

Halvorson noted that an ideal national health information system would: (1) be patient-centered and have continuity over time, staying with the patient, regardless of changes in provider, health plan, and geographic locale; and (2) make the right thing easy to do, by including systems that provide useful, timely reminders and instructions for patients and caregivers, so that together they can easily follow personalized health plans.

The Doctor of the Future
Victor S. Sierpina, University of Texas Medical Branch

Dr. Victor Sierpina's vision for integrative medicine includes the doctor of the future, who will be an integrative healer and whose practice differs in many ways from that of today's physician (Table 2-1). The doctor of the future will provide care that is patient centered and comprehensive (mind, body, and spirit), care that is both high-tech (using genomic prediction tools and systems biology, for example) and high-touch, and care that focuses on preventing disease and injury. The practice would be team based, and might include complementary and

TABLE 2-1 How the Doctor of the Future Will Function

The Care Process Is…..	The Doctor's Role Will Be…..
• Patient centered • Team based • High-touch, high-tech • Genomic and personalized • Preventive • Integrative	• A navigator • Part of a multidisciplinary team • Grounded in the community • Support social and environmental policies promoting health • Familiar with systems theory
And supports patients through….	And will follow….
• Complementary and alternative practices • Belief that the body helps heal itself	• Evidence-based, outcome-focused practices • Principles for creation of healing environments • The lead of empowered patients

alternative health practitioners, health coaches, and wellness mentors, as well as medical specialists. Putting the patient in the driver's seat allows representatives from any number of disciplines to serve as the navigator, helping people sort through conflicting data as well as many difficult choices they must make during their lifetimes. Finally, tomorrow's physicians would consistently assess new evidence to ensure that their practices meet the highest standards of quality and patient outcomes.

Sierpina noted that there is a certain tension between the body's capacity to heal itself, and the mechanical model in which doctors act as fixers. One goal of future practitioners may be to guide and empower patients toward self-healing. Consonant with this approach could be use of the full range of natural treatments that include attention to the mind and body, use of the safest and least expensive interventions first, and mobilizing community supports. This vision of the future doctor does not reflect a purely in-the-clinic model. Future clinicians, if they are to be integrative healers, need to be out where people are and participate in social and environmental policy change.

A focus on specific diseases and organ systems, rather than on overall health, results in part from an imbalance in the U.S. physician workforce, which is dominated by medical specialists. Meanwhile, primary care doctors are in short supply. The ratio of specialists to primary care doctors in the United States is roughly two to one (GAO, 2008), while in countries with universal access that ratio is inverted, with three primary care physicians for every specialist. Overreliance on specialty care moves in the opposite direction from the healers of the future described above. It leads to poorer patient outcomes and sharply increased health care costs: "Instead of spending a dollar for preventing problems, we spend $2 or $3 fixing them," Sierpina said.

He suggested the following four ways to counter this trend:

1. Change reimbursement policies to ensure that it is not more profitable to treat disease than to prevent it.
2. Enable the patient encounter to be long enough for clinicians to obtain sufficient information and provide adequate behavior-change counseling.
3. Expand the pool of primary care providers to include nurses, physician assistants, and other professional groups.
4. Create incentives for students to enter primary care and for medical schools to teach them.

Integrative Health and Cancer
Ellen L. Stovall, National Coalition for Cancer Survivorship

Patients with serious diseases and their families need easily accessible, high-quality information about their disease, its symptoms, and treatment alternatives and their side effects, said Ellen Stovall. In fact, 70 percent of patients with cancer seek such information. Yet, some of the largest, most frequently used search engines and websites make it difficult to find and access information on, for example, cancer and integrative medicine or cancer and complementary and alternative practices, even if the information is available on the site.

To the National Coalition for Cancer Survivorship, use of evidence-based medicine and evidence-based practices are basic quality indicators in cancer care. However, this usage is difficult to monitor in the face of the typically uncoordinated and unsystematic approaches to cancer care chronicled by a succession of IOM reports, including *From Cancer Patient to Cancer Survivor: Lost in Transition* (2005) and *Cancer Care for the Whole Patient: Meeting Psychosocial Health Needs* (2008). Some 95 percent of U.S. cancer patients are treated off protocol. "We have no idea what is happening to them, and that must change," Stovall said, adding that patients are being treated outside any system that places high priority on patient-centeredness, quality assurance, and accountability for providers' and health plans' treatment decisions. Halvorson's emphasis on treating each patient as a data point is therefore essential, she said.

Prime characteristics of patient-centered care involve attentively eliciting patient preferences and integrating mind, body, and spirit. However, cancer survivorship research reveals that when people are diagnosed with cancer, they temporarily lose the basic skills of everyday life. These include skills in communication, information seeking, decision making, problem solving, negotiation, and speaking up for their rights. These are necessary tools that all patients facing a serious illness need in order to be self-advocates over the course of treatment. Lack of these skills can inhibit formation of a mutual, trusting partnership between patient and doctor. Diagnosis of a serious disease represents a crisis that challenges the integration of mind, body, and spirit at a time when people must draw strength from all domains and need extraordinary support from trusted individuals.

Society embraces and emphasizes the race for the cure rather than the race for the care, said Stovall. The prevalent, laserlike focus on cure fails patients first and foremost—as well as everyone involved in their care—because cure may not be possible. Research involving three decades of cancer survivors indicates that more than death, survivors fear pain and suffering for themselves and their families. They also fear being abandoned by their physicians, reiterating the importance of keeping patients—not providers—at the center of the care process. In a truly patient-centered system, patients would never be abandoned and, for those who cannot be cured, the emphasis would shift to what *is* possible—healing.

Among the changes in the health system that would help patients with cancer and other serious conditions are greater acceptance and reimbursement of integrative health practices; reimbursement for the time health professionals spend with patients to focus on healing; having customized treatment and survivorship plans that clearly describe the goals of care for the whole patient, not merely the services intended to combat the disease; and using the process of creating the plan to build strong relationships among clinicians, patients, and families.

Communicating Health
Mehmet Oz, New York-Presbyterian Hospital/Columbia University
Medical Center

If much of Americans' health status depends on their personal behavior—whether it be smoking, dietary choices, exercise, or engaging appropriately with the health system—health professionals will need to communicate with patients much more effectively, in ways that are clear, motivating, and accessible, said Dr. Mehmet Oz.

Unfortunately, the current barrage of health-related communications that Americans receive often provides mixed messages, or incomplete, misleading, or out-of-context information. Even information derived from scientific studies can be confusing, such as conflicting information on the use of specific vitamins. In some cases, studies of issues the public cares about simply do not exist.

As use of integrative practices advances, health professionals may gain a deeper understanding of why some of these approaches work. However, Oz said that it may be very challenging in some cases to find hard evidence to present to the public about many of these approaches, or to support their broader use. There is often little or no funding to support the necessary research for integrative approaches to health. For the time being, the best test of whether doctors should recommend particular practices to their patients may be whether they would recommend them to their own families, said Oz.

The current medical system tends to focus on whether one intervention works better than another, while it almost never asks the question of whether a given intervention works better than doing nothing. Unfortunately, the latter is usually the question of concern to patients, said Oz. Patients want to know whether a recommended procedure is really necessary. Additionally, the current reimbursement structure encourages the use of expensive, sometimes invasive treatments over lifestyle changes, including nutrition and physical activity.

The concept of integrative health has a global component—not just because it sometimes uses traditional therapies from around the world, but also because of the mindset, endemic in many cultures around the world, that puts health and illness in a broad context and looks at the whole patient. In other words, it is patient centered. This contrasts with the U.S. health care system, in which clinicians take a problem-based approach. The lack of patient-centeredness in the system degrades trust between clinicians and their patients. A loss of trust, Oz said, is the primary ailment plaguing the whole system. "Suffering is not just about pain. Suffering is realizing you don't have control."

One way to increase patient control, Oz said, would be to create a "smart patient movement" that would empower patients to challenge certain assumptions about the therapies they are receiving or, more broadly, to participate in attempts to improve the health system. Such a movement would underscore the public's need to take more responsibility for personal health as well as provide opportunities to do so. The smart patient and integrative health movements must therefore develop and promote user-friendly ways for people to obtain health information that are easy to use and include positive, motivating messages.

Another way to increase patient control would be to encourage the use of health coaches and navigators. These important positions should be filled by knowledgeable people who can effectively guide and motivate patients to improve their health. Oz suggested that not all physicians have the time, the right expertise, or the interest in filling this role and that other professions should also be considered for it.

People make their health-related decisions in a social, economic, family, and cultural environment. A number of features of those environments need to change, in order to improve health. For example, U.S. agricultural and food enterprises produce 3,500 calories of food per person per day. The need to sell these products puts into play powerful marketing efforts that make it difficult for many Americans to maintain a moderate, healthy diet. It becomes nearly impossible to follow writer Michael Pollan's concise nutritional advice: "Eat food, not too much, mostly plants." Another environmental factor affecting health is the lack of opportunity for physical activity, which could include simple solutions, such as neighborhood sidewalks that would allow children to walk to school. A quick poll of the audience demonstrated that, as children, most audience members walked to school, yet few audience members' children do the same today. This demonstrated the fact that a few decades ago, half of American children walked to school, Oz said, compared to less than 10 percent today.

Finally, Oz suggested that a huge opportunity to improve the well-being of our nation would be to take advantage of the ServiceNation movement. Many service opportunities promote the health and well-being of citizens in need, the elderly, and children. High school graduates, retirees, and many others could—and already do—participate in community service through government-sponsored programs or through organizations like HealthCorps, which teaches children about diet, nutrition, and exercise.

Panel Discussion

Following the panel presentations, questions from the audience were submitted for further panel discussion, which was moderated by Johns.

Electronic Medical Records

One participant noted that some people have difficulty obtaining insurance coverage as a result of their medical history and the contents of their medical records, and queried whether such problems might be magnified if a national electronic health data system was created. Halvorson replied that universal insurance coverage will make it impossible to deny coverage for preexisting conditions. He noted that in Europe, where universal coverage is the norm, there is no health screening for insurance. He said this is also true for 95 percent of Americans who currently have access to coverage.

A corollary concern was raised regarding privacy protections for personal data in electronic health records. While there can be no absolute guarantee that an individual's medical record will be completely safe, Oz replied, in places such as British Columbia that have a national system for exchanging medical records, people find the advantages of the system outweigh their concerns about potential privacy breaches. Such a reaction might also occur among U.S. residents, except for those few with conditions that carry a real social stigma. Still, said Halvorson, "At the personal level we need to be absolutely bullet-proof on confidentiality issues," and this requires high standards, tough rules, and strong enforcement.

Integrative Medicine and Social Determinants of Health

Another participant asked how integrative medicine should address broad social factors such as social status, poverty, and education, which are important predictors of health status. Stovall responded by acknowledging the great disparities in the United States across many domains—

income, education, and health. Despite these disparities, she said, when patients receive care that is culturally appropriate and respects the values and norms of their community, they are more likely to follow their care plan and have better outcomes. In the long run, one approach to leveling the playing field in health care, she said, would be through the universal health care coverage that Halvorson endorsed.

Primary Care and Health Care Providers

Other questions probed whether caregivers other than physicians could provide some of the needed primary care. Panelists discussed options and noted that, while the health care workforce does need primary care physicians, it also needs geriatricians, nurse practitioners, physician assistants, and others who can provide primary care. Sierpina noted that health coaches and other intermediaries are also needed. Creating the right mix of professionals is one component of health reform, said Novelli.

Panelists further indicated that increasing the sheer numbers of new professionals may be necessary, but will not be sufficient. Without changing the fundamentals of the system, new professionals would only be able to do more of what is not working now, said Sierpina. He noted that the contributions of nurses, physician assistants, and many complementary professionals with long experience in prevention, primary care, and lifestyle issues could be increased. In addition, Halvorson said that tackling the problem of medical school debt might encourage more young physicians to enter the primary care field, even if it remains less remunerative than many specialties.

PRIORITY ASSESSMENT GROUP REPORT[1]

Integrative Medicine and Its Role in Shaping the National Health Reform Agenda

Dr. Reed Tuckson delivered the priority assessment group report, which focused on the health care reform agenda. This summary includes

---

[1]See Chapter 1 for a description of the priority assessment groups. Participants of this assessment group included Liza Goldblatt (moderator), Reed Tuckson (rapporteur) Susan Bauer-Wu, Jeffrey Bland, Sherman Cohn, Simon Fielding, Susan Folkman, Christy Mack, Diane Neimann, Margaret O'Kane, and Badri Rickhi.

the priorities discussed and presented by the assessment group to the plenary session for its discussion and consideration; these priorities do not represent a consensus or recommendations from the summit. The group advanced the following three top priorities.

The first priority identified by the group was the need to *advance a new and shared vision for health*—a national consensus that the health system should move away from the current predominant focus on the sickness model to a person-centered health, wellness, and prevention model that is holistic from birth to death, and involves individuals, families, and loved ones. It suggested that health care transformation should develop and build on a framework of individual responsibility for making responsible preventive and care choices that is supported by personally appropriate information and decision coaching. Promoting this vision for health requires consensus and a functional definition of integrative medicine that is easily understood and can be easily communicated. Additionally, the group also suggested a national campaign to inform important stakeholders about the shared vision for health and to more rapidly promote culture change.

The second priority is to *develop real evidence of the effectiveness of integrative health care*. This requires demonstration projects that move beyond a vision to evidence for effective models. These demonstration projects require two key features. First, the projects need to implement reimbursement models for disease prevention and health promotion that align and offer incentives for change. These include incentives for physicians to provide more cognitive interventions; incentives for patients to act on their own behalf and to use tools to help them follow recommended guidance; and incentives for providers to form teams that can offer more patient-centered, coordinated, and holistic care. Second, the demonstration projects must be designed to evaluate whether the integrative medicine models are cost-effective for short- and long-term care.

The third priority is to *develop the definition and criteria for evidence in integrative medicine*. To reflect integrative medicine's whole-person aims, this requires an understanding of the research questions attendant to moving from single episodic interventions to systems biology approaches and clusters of interventions. It also may require new standards of evidence for evaluation of quality and cost-effectiveness of outcomes.

The group identified several key actors and stakeholders whose involvement is necessary to advance the above priorities. Key actors and stakeholders identified include:

- purchasers and insurance plans;
- physicians, medical educators, and "environmental" physicians;
- other health professionals including behavioralists and
- sociologists;
- hospitals;
- pharmaceutical and technology companies;
- researchers, including the CDC and NIH;
- political leaders;
- education community;
- food industry; and
- community organizations, such as churches.

Finally, in response to the question of what goals are achievable in 3 years, the group concluded that significant progress will be marked by

- new initiatives, including demonstration projects that build on existing models of care and make good use of existing models, such as the Bravewell Collaborative clinical network sites, which provide a ready template for advancing innovations (These initiatives should include a diverse set of health care practitioners.);
- articulating the definition and vision of integrative medicine, gaining support from key constituencies, and launching the national campaign;
- active demonstration projects;
- progress in developing new evidence criteria;
- progress in reimbursement, especially because patient and physician incentives are already progressing in the marketplace that can be built upon; and
- advances in the integrative medicine agenda, as patients are "activated" to take control of disease prevention and management.

3

Models of Care

The keynote address for the session on models of care was provided by Dr. Donald Berwick, who emphasized the importance of design principles in model development and the necessity of patient-centeredness in all models intended to improve care. This panel discussion was moderated by Dr. Erminia Guarneri, Medical Director of the Scripps Center for Integrative Medicine, with panelists describing innovative models and necessary components for providing more integrative care, as well as the challenges they have faced.

Patient-centeredness was a key theme throughout this session. Berwick, for example, suggested that true patient-centeredness would attempt to explore patients' deep feelings about their health goals, so that care decisions would most effectively serve them. Panelists said that the disease-oriented approach of conventional allopathic medicine, described by Guarneri and Dr. Tracy Gaudet, does not establish the type of patient–clinician understanding Berwick and other participants described.

Constructive patient–provider relationships are essential to effectively providing preventive services to individuals with established chronic illnesses, as well as those without, Dr. Edward Wagner noted. He and others suggested that the mindset and principles of primary care may provide a sound foundation for integrative health care. Dr. Arnold Milstein analyzed components of small medical practices, where most physicians work, that are effective in developing teams to manage chronic diseases and control costs. His research emphasized, once again, the effectiveness of establishing relationships with patients and linking them to the care needed to address the behavioral and social elements of health care. This close management and use of established and innovative clinical tools, including web-based tools, are key features of integrative health practice, as described by Dr. David Katz, Dr. Mike Magee, and Gaudet. Demonstration studies of new models, especially those that include mechanisms of payment, could move integrative medicine forward and help overcome the current reimbursement challenges cited by Milstein, Katz, Gaudet, and Wagner.

MODELS KEYNOTE ADDRESS
Donald Berwick, Institute for Healthcare Improvement

In his remarks, Berwick, who leads the Institute for Healthcare Improvement, reflected on the array of earlier presentations and discussions, focusing on the elements of integration that emphasize patient-centeredness and smooth care transitions. He endorsed the Rorschach metaphor used earlier by Dr. Harvey Fineberg, saying that the speakers and audience were using a set of rather vaguely defined terms with great intention and wonderful spirit. However, he observed, these broad concepts of integrative medicine were being interpreted according to the individual backgrounds and needs of the participants. To make sense of the ambiguity around the terms and their usage, Berwick looked for the common purpose that pulled such diverse participants together, a purpose on which models of integrative medicine could be designed and built.

Despite the participants' enthusiastic support for integrative medicine, the simple notion of common purposes could prove to be a weak foundation for unity. The weakest foundation would be to unite based on a shared claim to a piece of a limited pie, said Berwick. A quest for greater reimbursement, for more payment for integrative care and alternative forms of care, may unite integrative medicine proponents today, but would soon divide them, as different groups assert their individual claims.

Professionals do need to be compensated for their services so that they can continue to carry out the work they love, he said. However, that goal is not a sufficient rallying point for building the cohesiveness necessary to advance integrative medicine. This movement must find a deeper offer to make to society. "Guilds are like mushrooms, and they will grow very fast before our eyes," he said. If integrative medicine becomes only a new list of guilds vying for reimbursement and organizational and professional power, "then we are wasting our time." Our health care system already has had too much negative experience with fragmentation, separation, and combat for a piece of the health care dollar. Thus, the first challenge for integrative care will be for the field to define what is being integrated, why, and then ultimately to integrate *itself.*

The Core Value: Patient-Centeredness

For nearly 20 years, committees of the Institute of Medicine have recommended better system designs in health care. These efforts have addressed traditional allopathic care, curative care, end-of-life care, and now the important new arena of integrative health care. This body of work is exemplified by IOM's quality of care initiatives that have included the Roundtable on Quality in the mid-1990s and the *Crossing the Quality Chasm* report in 2001, both of which Berwick participated in. These efforts also grappled with the question of underlying purpose: Should anything be better about American health care? If so, what should that be? The roundtable's answer emerged as a trio of generalizable problems: overuse, underuse, and misuse. It also developed a workable definition of quality: "The degree to which health services for individuals and populations increase the likelihood of desired health outcomes and are consistent with current professional knowledge."

The subsequent Committee on Quality of Health Care in America then built a framework for quality on the foundation developed by the roundtable. It went beyond overuse, underuse, and misuse to define a more ambitious agenda for the health care system. The committee concluded that, in order to achieve a system of excellence, the health system should have six goals: safety, effectiveness, patient-centeredness, timeliness, efficiency, and equity.

In the committee's early discussions, the list included patient control, rather than patient-centeredness. The change represented the tension and a compromise between those who thought health care should belong to the patient and those who thought patient decisions should be mediated by professionals who have knowledge and experience that patients do not possess. The term *patient-centeredness* was chosen to imply a partnership that includes dialog and shared control.

The committee also enumerated 10 rules to redesign health care processes. The third rule, titled "The patient as the source of control," says "Patients should be given the necessary information and the opportunity to exercise the degree of control they choose over health care decisions that affect them. The health system should be able to accommodate differences in patient preferences and encourage shared decision making." This backs away from the idea of patients' having total control, but supports the need for them to have the steering wheel in their hands. The committee's message was that patient-centeredness is important not only because it helps achieve better functional outcomes and greater safety, but that it is, in and of itself, *a property of good care.*

Other organizations—the Dartmouth Institute for Health Policy and Research, the Institute for Healthcare Improvement, and the Picker Institute, for example—began to expand the application of patient-centered care. The Picker Institute proposed that the very definition of quality lies through the patient's eyes. The Institute for Healthcare Improvement asks patients whether they can agree with the statement that their provider—whether it be physician, practice, or hospital—gives them "exactly the help I want and need, exactly when I want and need it," which delegates the very definition of excellence to the experience of the person served.

This is a high standard, but one deemed necessary in almost every other consumer industry. Modern health care did not begin with a patient-centered standard. Instead, the field remained rooted in concepts proposed by Eliot Freidson in the mid-1900s. Freidson theorized that professions like medicine reserve to themselves the authority to judge the quality of their own work. Society gives professionals that authority on the assumption that the profession will be altruistic, has knowledge the public does not and cannot have, and can regulate itself. Again, this is not the basis for consumer relationships in most other industries.

Berwick described how the model of patient-centeredness is being translated into practice in various settings—Mayo Clinic's emphasis on "the needs of the patient come first," or the statement that Boston's Parker Hill Hospital set above its door, authored by its CEO, Arthur Berarducci, "Every Patient is the Only Patient," or creation of the healing environments envisioned in the Planetree model of care. New work at the Institute for Healthcare Improvement focuses on three population-based views of excellence, constituting the so-called "Triple Aim"—judging the experience of care through the patient's eyes, addressing the health of the population served, and considering per capita cost as a measure of system quality.

Prior to recent decades and in many cultures worldwide, the dominant definition of health was, in essence, the extent to which the body can heal itself—physically, mentally and spiritually. In this view, the role of medicine and health care is that of a servant, an assistant to bodily processes already under way. Its job "is to let [the body] do so, to stand out of the way, and to offer resources or assets to allow [healing] to move forward," said Berwick. This conception adds to the significance of the patient-centeredness concept and begins to suggest what integrative medicine could mean and what its purpose is.

Achieving Integrative Medicine's Aims

Just as the IOM committee on quality defined a set of design principles that could realize its vision of quality care, certain design principles might move the health system toward more integrative care—"the care that connects technology to souls." Berwick shared a poignant personal anecdote that illustrated the ways in which right care needs to draw from the integration of personal values and priorities with clinical concerns. Drawing on the day's discussion, Berwick suggested eight such principles, summarized in Box 3-1.

The first principle put forward was to *put the patient at the center*. Good examples of this are the chronic care model developed by Wagner, or the Mayo Clinic's "the needs of the patients come first."

Second, and related, is *individualization*. New technology, such as advances in genomics, makes the individualization of care ever more possible. Berwick predicted that a science-based, individually focused, predictive system of health and care could be the death knell for insurance as we know it today. Actuarial prediction of costs becomes impossible when "every patient is the only patient" and care is customized to the level of the individual.

BOX 3-1
Berwick's Principles for Integrative Medicine

1. Place the patient at the center.
2. Individualize care.
3. Welcome family and loved ones.
4. Maximize healing influences within care.
5. Maximize healing influences outside care.
6. Rely on sophisticated, disciplined evidence.
7. Use all relevant capacities—waste nothing.
8. Connect helping influences with each other.

Third, *welcome and embrace* the patient's family, loved ones, and community. This means not separating a person from the loving community that provides energy, self-esteem, solace, and wisdom. In today's hospitals, "We create nothing so reliably as we create loneliness," said Berwick. New Zealand's Maori health care system defines health quality as including physical health, emotional health, spiritual health, and family health. Such a definition emphasizes the essential value of connectedness.

Fourth, *maximize healing influences in health care facilities.* In other words, make current treatment facilities healing places by, for example, refocusing human interactions and using evidence-based designs that reduce patient, family, and staff stress; prevent errors and nosocomial infections; and increase positive influences on health status.

Fifth, *maximize healing influences outside the care system.* This requires the system and providers to learn about and help patients implement the many actions they can take in their daily lives to heal themselves or minimize the impact of illness or disability. The formal system of care rarely considers these opportunities.

Sixth, *rely on sophisticated and disciplined evidence.* For an integrative system of care, this may be the most difficult challenge. It requires forms of evidence and approaches to learning that are far less developed and far less recognized today than canonical experimental designs and randomized trials. This is because, in the full expression of patient-centered, individualized, integrative care, each person is a continuous experiment of one, and rigorous measurement and evaluation need to be applied to individual learning cycles, over the long term. This type of research is not currently embraced by traditional research funders or scientific journals, Berwick noted. While patient-centered research needs to be every bit as robust and disciplined as current methods, it requires a forward leap in methodology to learn from the experience of the individual patient.

Seven, *use all relevant capacities.* In a sense, the potential health care workforce is exactly as large as the entire population. The concept that we have a shortage in primary care is conditioned on a very limited view of the capacity of almost all human beings, said Berwick. Individual patients, their families, and even their community can have insights about the person's condition that formal care providers cannot.

Finally, *the importance of connection.* Potential helping influences must connect with one another. One strategy for this is through health navigators and health coaches. Another is through interconnected information systems. However, the fundamental generator of connection begins with an attitude of cooperation among all individuals and institutions involved in a person's care.

Conclusions

Durable, worthy connections among and across the many individuals and organizations supporting integrative medicine can be forged by rediscovering and affirming a common purpose: *what we wish to heal.* What we health care professionals wish to heal, Berwick suggested, are those who come to us for help; ourselves who are among them; a broken, imbalanced, greedy, technocentric, unself-conscious health care system; and a world that has displayed infinite cleverness in increasing human suffering. "The sources of suffering are in separateness," Berwick said, "and the remedy is in remembering that we are in this together. Integration, if it is to thrive, is the name of a duty to contribute what we can to a troubled and suffering planet."

PANEL ON MODELS OF CARE

Panel Introduction
Erminia Guarneri, Scripps Center for Integrative Medicine
Panel Moderator

Dr. Erminia Guarneri described how, when she graduated from medical school in 1988, she thought that she knew everything there was to know about medicine after reading the essential textbooks of the field. As a young intern and resident, she was rewarded for applying the find-it-and-fix-it approach, getting her differential diagnoses right, followed by appropriate patient treatment and discharge. That was considered a success, and she was considered a good physician because she could achieve it. In those terms she again proved successful in the mid-1990s, this time in the field of coronary stenting. She—and the field—said that correctly placed and correctly timed stents could wipe out heart disease, the number one killer of Americans today.

For Guarneri, the wake-up call came when she realized that "a 16-millimeter stent does not prevent cardiovascular disease." Nor does commonly used statin therapy, which only reduces morbidity and mortality by about 30 percent. Further, she was learning from her patients that, when it comes to cardiovascular health, the illnesses of loneliness, depression, anger, and hostility are every bit as devastating as hypertension and diabetes. The wake-up call told her that "we need to embrace it all"—the best of what she had learned in medical school, the best of a wide array of therapies, and the best of high technology, all blended with a recognition that the complex human being is made up of body, mind, emotions, and spirit. "It is a misnomer to think that clinicians can just treat the physical body and call it medicine," said Guarneri.

For the past 12 years, Guarneri has been working on a model of care that embraces the fact that having a positive purpose in life is as important as good laboratory values and that our social and physical environment is as important as having a low LDL reading.

Models That Integrate Continuous Care
Across Caregivers and Settings
Edward Wagner, MacColl Institute for Healthcare Innovation
at Group Health Center for Health Studies

Dr. Edward Wagner raised several particularly challenging issues for integrative care. Earlier summit discussions highlighted the unsound state of primary care in the United States. Yet Wagner noted that primary care has the mindset, the orientation, and the relationship with the population that make it a promising foundation for integrative health care. Since it is not realistic or desirable to expect the development of an entirely separate integrated health care system, it is necessary to update primary care as it exists today, in order to make it an effective platform for building integrative care models.

Wagner's second point related to the false distinction commonly drawn between preventive care and care for chronic illnesses and conditions. This distinction must be broken down, he said, because the needs of the healthy population and the needs of the vast majority of those who have chronic disorders—some 40 to 50 percent of the population—are, in many cases, the same. Like those without chronic disease, people with chronic conditions still require prevention efforts for conditions they do not have. At the same time, prevention of adverse events is also required for the condition or conditions they *do* have.

Both groups need effective, evidence-based clinical, behavioral, and supportive treatments. Fortunately, the health system has made great progress in this arena, and such treatments now exist. Both groups need meaningful, personalized information, and they need emotional and psychosocial support to help them in their self-care and self-management. Both groups also need regular assessments tailored to the severity of their individual risks or health condition, systematic follow-up, and coordination of services across care settings.

Over the past two or three decades, researchers and quality improvement professionals have begun to understand the system changes that assure that these needs are met. Reviews of interventions across a multitude of conditions and situations show that effective practice changes are similar, whether in the preventive or in the chronic care management arena. Such interventions involve greater use of nonphysician members of integrated, high-functioning practice teams. They also include planned, organized patient encounters. For prevention services, encounters may be organized around protocols, such as those developed for prenatal or well-child care. These protocols, for example, involve giving parents an active role in managing their children's health or medical conditions. Evidence-based protocols, which have been developed not only for children, can easily be translated into checklists, e-prescribing, and follow-up steps that assure that the right thing to do is the default. More intensive management is necessary for people at high risk, but information technology can facilitate the planning and organization of their care, too.

Fulfilling patient needs and achieving system change for prevention is where primary care comes in. Primary care needs to be transformed into a more effective foundation for integrative health care, through wider implementation of the kinds of practice teams and improved patient encounters described. "The future of our health care system depends on primary care's ability to improve the quality and efficiency of its preventive and chronic illness care," Wagner said.

Wagner noted that improving efficiency begins with clear policies about which interventions are of value, which are uncertain yet safe—and their use, therefore, subject to personal preference—and which are ineffective or unsafe. Clarity about the performance of various interventions will make the development of high-quality, efficient primary care easier. Additionally, more time, energy, and perhaps more people on the primary care team than the current reimbursement system allows are required for primary care personnel to achieve the ideal of timely, person-centered, continuous, and coordinated care. Payment reform and information technology can help a great deal, but to enable primary care to meet the goals of integrative medicine requires a major transformation and redesign of primary care practice, he said.

Care Models That Lower Per Capita Spending and Improve Outcomes
Arnold Milstein, Pacific Group on Health and Mercer Health & Benefits

The current top national health care policy priority is to reduce near-term per capita health care spending, or to at least reduce its rate of growth. According to Milstein this needs to be accomplished in a way that is clinically responsible, by preserving or, ideally, improving both patient experience and clinical outcomes. He indicated that much integrative medicine emphasizes upstream care and long-term benefits, which does not position it well to reduce near-term spending. Milstein explored the question of whether integrative medicine could play a role in reducing near-term spending, noting that the national policy priority to reduce spending is especially important for families in the bottom half of America's income distribution, who are unable to afford conventional health insurance, but not poor enough to qualify for Medicaid.

Working with several insurers across the nation, Milstein identified five physician practices that have successfully used integrative care methods to achieve positive patient experience ratings, improve clinical outcomes, *and* reduce short-term costs by at least 15 percent per patient, per year—his cutoff point for including a practice in his onsite study.

No large integrated health care delivery systems were able to achieve this trio of accomplishments. This does not mean that large high-performing systems do not exist, just that they did not emerge in this search. (He noted that most observers believe that large systems have the greatest potential for improvement in all six aims of quality health care defined by the IOM's *Crossing the Quality Chasm* report [IOM, 2001a]). Milstein theorized that "smaller organizations may be more agile in cutting-edge attempts to break through the price-performance frontier."

The five successful practice settings Milstein identified were of two types. The first model was "needs-tailored." These practices redesigned their care platform to address shared needs of chronic illness patients. They were the types of practices that Wagner described during his presentation.

The second successful model was a somewhat larger practice, containing about 60 predominantly primary care physicians. This group had gone one step further and developed multiple distinct care platforms to address subcategories of need among chronic illness patients. These were not only disease-specific platforms; some were built to respond to narrow problems that cut across diagnoses, such as presurgical stabilization. Leadership for these platforms was provided by hospitalists, but they were mostly implemented by a nonphysician team that included nutritionists, ambulatory care nurses, and a variety of other health professions. Hospitalists led the teams because they are the clinicians most often face to face with the failures of the ambulatory care system.

Both models depended heavily on their health plans' sharing with them the savings achieved from their improved care delivery methods. None of the practices could have survived on current fee-for-service payments. Almost all of them tried to be globally capitated for as many of their patients as possible, because their better methods of caring for high-risk patients are simply financially infeasible with the very brief encounters allowed under current fee-for-service reimbursement rules.

Milstein thinks of these five practice settings as "medical home runs." They achieved positive clinical outcomes and patient experiences, and they reduced total health care spending. A reengineered care model allowed them to reduce, cost-effectively, the number of expensive health crises among their chronic disease patients. Three principal strategies helped them accomplish this.

First, the practices excel at salient chronic illness *caring*. Their physicians and care teams effectively convey to patients that it matters to them personally that the patient be spared health crises. This has a highly favorable effect on patient self-management and provides a sense of hope. Second, they use teams effectively. Third, each practice discerned that selected specialists in their communities exemplify high-quality, conservative practice, and they were careful to refer patients only to these specialists or to other similarly conservative service providers, such as pain management centers.

In most cases, the successful practices incorporated many features of integrative health care by routinely assessing psychological, social, and environmental health risk factors for unstable patients. To enable this, the practices allowed at least 30 minutes for each clinical encounter, during which time clinicians thoroughly reviewed the patient's list of problems. After this review, instead of "reaching for the doorknob," as Milstein put it, providers would ask, "What else is bothering you?" and "What is happening in your life?" The providers took the time to understand the patients. This parallels the in-depth understanding of patients urged by Berwick.

The practices are prepared to act swiftly and effectively on psychosocial problems they uncover. The physician-supervised psychosocial SWAT team comprises a nurse, social worker, and community health worker. It also has an attorney available to handle relevant legal situations.

Psychological, social, and environmental objectives are included in patient care plans. An example of such integrative care design was found in a gym that one practice set up for seniors who needed strength and balance training. In most gyms, the forward-facing exercise bicycles make workouts solitary and boring. By contrast, in this gym, low-noise exercycles were arranged in a circle to give users a chance to converse with five other people while getting their exercise. Such an integrative care design increased patients' willingness to work out and strengthened their social networks, which conferred additional health benefits.

A final integrative strategy that these successful practices employed was use of a thorough "failure mode analysis" of unplanned hospitalizations. Whenever one occurs, staff members probe for its root causes and work to fix whatever is necessary to prevent future hospitalizations—even when the causes involve factors or remedies outside the boundaries of conventional care, such as finding summer air-conditioning for a home-bound patient with COPD.

Models That Promote Health, Wellness, and Preventions
David L. Katz, Prevention Research Center,
Yale University and the Integrative Medicine Center,
Griffin Hospital

Two forceful currents in modern patient care are the primacy of the patient and the primacy of scientific evidence. These currents often flow in opposition and, when they collide, they produce very turbulent and troubled waters. Evidence-based integrative medicine may be the best way to assure that patients are not left at the water's edge, with no good way to obtain relief, said Katz.

Katz, an internist and preventive medicine specialist at the Integrative Medicine Center at Griffin Hospital in Derby, Connecticut, described the Center's model of integrative medicine, which includes a holistic, team-based approach to caring for patients. Like the other conventionally trained physicians at the center, he works side by side with naturopathic physicians and in close collaboration with an array of colleagues from the various disciplines of alternative care.

When a new patient comes to the center, both the conventionally trained and naturopathic physicians see the patient and conduct an evaluation. They immediately confer and share their recommendations across a broad spectrum of options. This model of care attracts so-called difficult patients who have "been everywhere, tried everything, and simply aren't better," said Katz. One of the most compelling arguments for the integration of care, Katz said, is that, for such patients, the only alternative to integrative approaches "is the disintegration of care, leaving them to shuffle around aimlessly in the pursuit of the one thing they want—to be well." The center's premise is that differently trained practitioners can offer better patient guidance and better navigation by working together.

Katz said that standards of evidence, particularly the reliance on evidence from randomized controlled trials, are applied too rigidly to patient care. For example, the results of a trial may not directly pertain to an individual patient, and it may be difficult to assess the extent to which the results *are* relevant. Even when a patient's characteristics suggest a correspondence with effective treatments indicated by trials, many patients are still not helped. He supports a more thoughtful application of evidence that considers effectiveness, safety, and the level and quality of scientific support. Using this standard, center staff considers various ways to treat the presenting problem or constellation of problems, taking patient preferences into account.

Clinicians are often in a gray zone in deciding among competing treatment approaches, particularly when caring for a patient who has not been helped by conventional therapies. When faced with the needs of a patient not met by the best-studied modalities, the only choices physicians have are to leave patients to sort things out on their own, or to help them choose among the less-studied alternatives. It is at just such times that the expertise of the clinician is most needed, said Katz, to help identify the most rational next choice, based on considerations of probable effectiveness and safety.

The center's integrative care model can be applied across the spectrum of prevention: primary prevention, which includes health promotion and specific defenses against disease; secondary prevention, which includes early detection and management to prevent progression of diseases and their symptoms; and tertiary prevention, which reduces the problems associated with an established disease or injury.

Katz illustrated the center's work with brief reports of two clinical cases. He used these examples to demonstrate how integrative, holistic, team-based approaches can be used to successfully diagnose and treat patients who had not experienced improved outcomes through the conventional medical system. Katz noted that holistic practice helps clinicians find ways to reconcile responsible use of science and responsiveness to the needs of patients. These needs continue, even when evidence runs thin. It should not be necessary to choose between the two. The aspiration of a more holistic and integrative care system is meritorious and worthy, said Katz. Getting there may not be easy, but "we should certainly persevere."

Models That Optimize Health and Healing
Across the Life Span
Tracy Gaudet, Duke Integrative Medicine

Keying off the day's presentations and the development of innovative models for integrative care in the United States and elsewhere, Gaudet described a vision for a transformed health care system and how the models might be achieved within it. The changes needed are not incremental; they require a complete revolution in the mindset that shapes our current system, said Gaudet.

Chronic conditions account for more than 75 percent of U.S. health care costs or approximately $1.87 trillion per year. The development and consequences of chronic conditions are heavily influenced by individuals' lifestyle choices and health behavior. Making a difference in these trends will require a true health care recovery plan. Increasingly, there is both a professional *and* an economic imperative for change.

Gaudet noted that the current health care model does not work because it starts from the wrong place. It is problem based and disease oriented, and it inadequately addresses the significance of personal health behavior in maintaining health and preventing disease. Unless health care professionals can help patients understand their sense of meaning and purpose and the sources of joy in their life, people do not alter their lifestyle choices or modify their health behavior. Nor will behavior changes be sustainable unless they have deep personal significance, she said.

No aspect of the current health care system is actually designed to address the personal needs of the individual, and this is the fundamental organizational mindset that must change, according to Gaudet. If clinicians understand this concept deeply, they will recognize they must start their relationship with their patient from an entirely new place. While the underlying concept is radical, she said, its implementation can be accomplished relatively easily within current structures.

Gaudet suggested that four primary strategies would create a new framework for health. The first strategy is the creation of new standardized tools for clinical use. In the current medical model, physicians have tools that guide them in taking histories and performing physical exams. These problem-based tools start with the chief complaint. A new integrative intake tool that asks about and addresses all aspects of a patient's health would reorient the patient–physician partnership from the outset. Instead of a disease-based medical record, clinicians would use a whole-person medical record that reflects the physical, mental, spiritual, and relationship-centered life of a patient. Instead of creating a problem list, they would develop an integrative health risk assessment. Finally, instead of this resulting in an assessment and plan for the *problem*, clinicians would create a health profile and a personalized health plan for the *person*. Tools like these would help clinicians look at the individual's health risk from a holistic perspective and lay out a path for moving toward optimal health.

The second strategy Gaudet discussed would be the development of strong provider teams that are not necessarily centered around a physician. Important roles and functions are missing from today's conventional medical teams. One discipline that is critical to this approach to health is the integrative health coach who would fill a currently unmet need in the system: a professionally trained provider whose expertise is in partnering with patients to help them enact the lifestyle changes and behavior that result in better health.

Third, training in the health care disciplines must be geared to teaching the core competencies needed to deliver this model of health. Reoriented educational programs are needed for existing disciplines and providers, as well as new programs that would prepare new members of the health care team.

Finally, Gaudet suggested that efforts should be made to disseminate and implement new models of care that are emerging, for example, from the Bravewell Clinical Network. The centennial of the last major reform in medical education and health care is approaching; the "Flexner Report" (1910) brought stronger science into medical education, and the reorganization of the Johns Hopkins School of Medicine served as the demonstration project for that initiative. No matter how insightful and powerful Flexner's report was, Gaudet said that if it had not been paired with a demonstration project, its impact most likely would have been minimal. The time is now for a new vision for 21st century health care. A clearly articulated vision, combined with a strong demonstration project, can catalyze the second revolution in health care.

Models That Promote Primary Care, Medical Homes, and Patient-Centered Care
Mike Magee, Center for Aging Services Technologies, American Association of Homes & Services for the Aging

Past work on cross-sector partnerships and the elements that make them successful may cast light on some of the requirements for moving forward with integrative medicine. Magee has studied such partnerships and finds them analogous to the situation confronted by the multiple disciplines that integrative health care requires.

In the beginning, such partnerships focus on developing a common language and tools and articulating a common mission and values. These needs are important preliminary steps to assure sustainability and success. However, in the long run, three critical elements determine whether cross-sector partnerships thrive, said Magee. These elements can be expressed by how effectively partnerships answer these key questions: Do you know what you want to build? Is the vision sufficiently powered not to be overtaken by change? Is there readiness to build out that vision? Over time, the supporters of integrative health care will need to answer the questions.

A decades-long supporter of relationship-based health care, Magee agrees with the values embedded in the current medical home concept endorsed by various medical and osteopathic professional organizations. It emphasizes comprehensive partnerships, mutual decision-making teams, holistic coordination, facilitated technology, quality, safety, evidence, access, and personal relationships. These are worthy attributes, he said, but the medical home concept may be significantly underpowered to manage the nation's future health needs. His concerns begin at the starting point for care and can be summarized in six words: "Too much medical, not enough home."

A home-centered health care model would focus on helping people achieve their full human potential. This model requires looking at the many forces and individuals that influence health-related decisions day by day, month after month. For a young child, the view may extend out over a 100-year horizon. Magee said that it requires planning ahead, considering a person's uniqueness, socially and scientifically. It requires "being where the person lives," in the home.

In this context, *home* means both a geographic and a virtual place. It is where one feels safe and secure, supported and loved, awash in social capital. While the geographic home may change location, the state of feeling at home should ideally follow. "So much has changed all around us that perhaps we could be excused for having overlooked the home as a logical destination and cornerstone for the health system," said Magee. Misreading the significance of trends has compounded the problem.

Magee noted three examples of trends that affect home and family that health care systems should address: how longevity has made families more complex, as they have moved from involving three generations to four- and five-generations; how the Internet, which can push massive amounts of information at high rates of speed, is essentially geography free and offers almost infinite opportunities for connection; and how three decades of consumer health information has led to empowerment that has suppressed medical paternalism and encouraged teams and mutual decision making.

This last trend is now giving way to health activism, led primarily by informal family caregivers. Magee said that most of these are middle-aged women, often managing frailty in the older generation and immaturity in the younger. Caregivers labor as both providers and consumers, yet are not generally recognized as part of the health care team. For them, it is not the lack of information that is literally killing them, it is the lack of a system.

A sufficiently powered vision of a home-centered health care model must make complexity, connectivity, and consumerism an advantage. However, our health care system continues to focus on the loop from the doctor's office to the hospital and back again as shown in Figure 3-1. The home, if considered at all, is an afterthought. A person with a health concern must find a way into the loop.

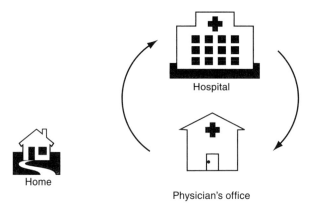

FIGURE 3-1 Doctor–hospital loop.

Magee suggested a new health care system where the home is at the center, and the loop begins from home and goes to the care team and back to the home as shown in Figure 3-2. A rich array of information that is personalized and customized with vital signs, diagnostics, and planning milestones could be transmitted automatically and wirelessly from the home to the care team. In the other direction, data, analysis, advice, support, and coaching could come into the home continuously. All would be part of a virtual system committed to efficiency, connectivity, and mobility, rather than being tied to the bricks and mortar of health care facilities. Such a vision obviously entails serious challenges, but it builds on a number of our strengths.

Magee highlighted five examples of strengths that could be built upon. The first strength is the high value that Americans place on their homes, where loved ones support and value them. "Americans abhor homelessness yet have learned to accept healthlessness," he said.

The second strength is Americans' increasing support for universal health care. With this right must come responsibility, he said. Readiness to define roles and responsibilities in individuals, families, and communities in return for universal care could provide multiple societal benefits.

Third, health care providers are beginning to accept information technology. The next step will be to take full advantage of its capacity to humanize, plan, connect, and bring order and sense to a segmented and broken system. Helpful resources for expanding this capacity might be

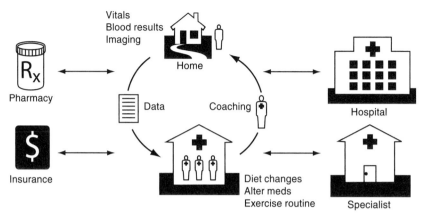

FIGURE 3-2 Home-centered care team loop.

found by partnering with sectors that have tremendous information technology expertise and an existing position in the home but which are currently locked out of health care, like the financial, home technology, and home entertainment sectors.

Fourth, many people are beginning to appreciate that, rather than creating a socioeconomic digital divide, information technology may do just the opposite. Connectivity can be targeted first at those who need it most, whether that is an 18-year-old pregnant, single mother of two in West Philadelphia; a Montana farm family 200 miles from the nearest hospital; or the only daughter of a widowed mother living three states away.

Finally, embracing these trends may allow more efficient and effective management of the existing chronic disease burden while simultaneously building a truly preventive system that will serve generations to come.

The missing connection at this point is a software application, which Magee predicts will be ubiquitous on all new computers within 5 years. This application should be called a "lifespan planning record (LPR)". LPRs will supplant personal health records and will come from the consumer side—with or without the support of clinicians. LPRs could be the tipping point enabling a truly preventive health care system. They will be a graphically pleasing, highly-powered application capable of automatically extracting and compiling a wide range of individual, family, community, environmental, and scientific data, then converting that data into a personalized, predictive, preventive, and participatory strategic health plan. LPRs will accept real-time modifications and provide information and support for plan adherence. With what we currently know, the 100-year plan for today's child could already be imbedded with thousands of targeted inputs, he said, and 10 years from now, that plan could include hundreds of thousands of data points.

In short, Magee said that the medical home movement's values are not wrong, but its destination is, and that must change. Preserving relationship-based health care requires embracing current trends and leading with a vision sufficiently powerful to excite the imagination. This vision must embrace complexity, connectivity, and consumerism, while reinforcing the social health capital imbedded in relationships between people and the people who are taking care of them.

Panel Discussion

Following the panel presentations, the audience submitted questions for further panel discussion, which was moderated by Guarneri.

Reimbursement

The first question asked about the reasons that many young physicians choose to go into specialty care. These reasons are not all financial and include perceptions about intellectual challenges and professional respect. Ed Wagner responded that nonfinancial disincentives are powerful, but that the lack of respect is largely evident by the way primary care physicians are paid. He said that the most important way to overcome the payment problem would be to stop reimbursing primary care physicians using the fee-for-service payment model. Fee-for-service has a variety of disincentives to providing the kind of personalized, integrated care discussed at the summit. These disincentives are not just the levels of reimbursement, but the emphasis that the fee-for-service system places on throughput and brief interactions. "If we can do any one thing in health care reform, I would say get primary care on capitation as quickly as possible," Wagner said.

Noting that reimbursement ran through much of the dialogue, Katz said, "We have not so much an evidence-based system of health care as a reimbursement-based system of health care." For example, the reimbursement system makes it difficult to provide team care. If every patient sees not just one high-cost clinician but several simultaneously, the costs are prohibitive. Demonstration research programs are needed to test the effectiveness of team-based practice, said Katz.

A program designed by Dean Ornish, in which Guarneri participated many years ago, showed that every dollar spent on care for very sick cardiac patients could save $6.66 on angioplasty and bypass surgery. Thus there are precedents for demonstration models and clinical networks that can deliver effective preventive care. We should test these concepts and take them out of the realm of integrative medicine, she suggested, saying, "Let's just make it medicine."

Genomics and Epigenomics

Another participant asked about the role that emerging concepts within systems biology that relate to genomics, proteonomics, and metabolomics will play in integrative medicine in the future.

Certainly, Guarneri said, we will have people rushing to websites like 23andMe and Navigenics to have a look at their genomes. They will obtain the information, but they may not realize that genetic risk does not mean they will manifest a particular disease. Their genetic blueprint can be influenced by their environment through epigenetic processes. Integrative medicine includes attention to the environment, where and how people live, with whom they live, and their lifestyle—what they eat and how they exercise, for example. Understanding these factors, as well as the biologic ones, is essential to unfolding the potential for illness. After all, "we are more than our genes," she said.

Katz added, "As we pursue the trees represented by our genetic polymorphisms, we ought not lose sight of the forest." The overwhelming contribution of personal behavior to morbidity and mortality has been well elucidated for nearly 20 years. Health care providers should focus at least as much on applying the knowledge they already have, he said, "which does not require the use of electron microscopes or profiling our individual genomes." If they did, they could slash heart disease by as much as 80 percent, diabetes by 90 percent, and cancer by 60 percent or more. While it will be helpful to know what specific genetic variations an individual has, there is an enormous wellspring of opportunity already in place that practitioners should not overlook as they attempt to foresee future events.

Strategically, it may be wise to link integrative health to these technological advances in a profound way, said Gaudet. She said "We need a health care system, not a disease care system, if we are going to utilize the science that we are advancing." While people may believe high-tech interventions are at the opposite end of the spectrum from integrative health, she said, high-tech interventions need to be incorporated into integrative health care in the same personalized and holistic way as other services.

PRIORITY ASSESSMENT GROUP REPORT[1]

Identifying and Advancing Workable Models of Integrative Care

Themes and Highlights

Dr. Fred Sanfilippo provided the report for the priority assessment group that reviewed ways to promote models of integrative care. This summary reflects the priorities discussed and presented by the assessment group to the plenary for its discussion and consideration; these priorities do not represent a consensus or recommendations from the Summit. This group began with the presumption that its discussion would focus on models that represented substantial changes, and it discussed priorities, relevant actors, and short- and long-term progress.

The group's three most important priorities were that models should demonstrate value, sustainability, and scalability. In discussing ways to demonstrate value, the group acknowledged that all models have *potential* value of one type or another. Prime indicators of a model's value are whether it achieves quality outcomes and is safe; another is reflected in its costs relative to these outcomes; and another is whether it effectively engages patients and, in their eyes, provides satisfactory care.

In terms of sustainability, the group noted that models being assessed must work across populations, be financially viable and self-sustaining, and self-actualizing or continually improving. To the group, scalability meant making sure that the models could scale up to large and more diverse populations, but also scale down to the individual level. The

---

[1]See Chapter 1 for a description of the priority assessment groups. Participants of this assessment group included Carol Black (moderator), Fred Sanfilippo (rapporteur), Brian Berman, Lilian Cheung, Mary Hardy, Mark Hyman, Bradly Jacobs, Woodson Merrell, Chuck Sawyer, Timothy Birdsall, and Lori Knutson.

models should work effectively across providers and employers and across communities and states.

The second question the group addressed related to key actors and their roles. People who are recipients of health care services were deemed the most important group of actors. Their roles include becoming more aware of nonmedical factors that affect health and healing, including social, economic, environmental and behavioral factors; setting realistic expectations for their care; and demanding changes and accountability from payers and providers. The second set of key actors identified is the health care provider group. Their role is to be proactive, not reactive, and to develop comprehensive, coordinated models of health care delivery that involve multidisciplinary teams whose membership reflects patient needs. These teams should take into account both biological and nonbiological contributors to illness, health, and healing. A third set of key actors comprises facilitators—employers, state and federal governments, payers, and others whose role is to help drive this change by demanding value. Another group of actors is found in academia, where educational programs can foster this broader approach to health and healing. Such programs should be located in each of the health care disciplines and professions, and new programs can create new disciplines that may be needed, such as coaches, navigators, and others.

The group noted that even within 3 years, it should be possible to have the evidence to identify some demonstration models that work, as well as some well-functioning, vertically and horizontally integrated delivery systems. It would be important to demonstrate, in this time, successful ways to provide financial incentives for developing these models and rewarding their development. Finally, in 3 years, there should be good evidence of changes in the educational curricula for existing disciplines but also educational programs for new professional categories.

In 10 years, the group said that it should be possible to identify best-practice models that fulfill the value parameters described earlier. These models should be supported by reformed financial and reimbursement systems for health care; this step is necessary for any of the advancement of integrative medicine in general. By 10 years time, information technology applications should be in place that can facilitate health care transactions and provide decision support. Also by 10 years time, and with the right education, both the public and providers can be expected to have a much better understanding of the socioeconomic factors in health and disease and should have begun to address them.

The group also identified several major next steps. The first steps are to create a definition of integrative health care that engenders wide agreement and then to reach agreement on a standardized set of outcome measures. Next would be to inventory existing models and identify their pluses and minuses; to inventory the health provider arrangements that exist in various models and see how they might fit into a more coherent model or inform the future; and to inventory data and information systems to gain a comprehensive view of current best practices and effectiveness around work processes and decision support. Other important steps the group suggested would be for the Centers for Medicare and Medicaid Services to support demonstration projects, the National Institutes of Health to support clinical effectiveness studies, and the IOM to hold follow-up summits.

Discussion and Questions

The summit participants' discussion of the assessment group report revealed a number of models that could be ripe subjects for demonstration projects in integrative medicine almost immediately, if funding for such studies were available. According to Sanfilippo, applications for such funding might come from a variety of places, including large employers and various communities positioned to move ahead fairly quickly. Some existing projects with potential to participate in a trial that might not immediately be thought of as integrative care models also were suggested, such as the life program of the University of Pennsylvania's School of Nursing, which is a capitated, independent living program for elders that involves nurses, doctors, dentists, and occupational and physical therapists.

Another audience member cautioned against assuming more empowerment and health literacy than many people actually have. The participant noted that any demonstration model would be a helpful advance, especially if it included facilitators, health care advocates, language interpreters, and information technology specialists who could make care more accessible to everyone.

4

Science

Science is nothing but trained and organized common sense.
—Thomas H. Huxley

The keynote address for the session on science was delivered by Dr. Dean Ornish. Ornish surveyed the key fields related to integrative medicine, providing examples of the effectiveness of integrative interventions in improving patients' health. The panel discussion was moderated by Dr. Bruce McEwen of the Rockefeller University, with panelists offering their perspectives and priorities surrounding the development and advancement of the evidence base for integrative medicine.

Topics reviewed focused on the complex interplay of biology, behavior, psychosocial factors, and environment shaping health and disease. Often, as Ornish pointed out, these interactions can produce synergistic results—for good or ill. This very complexity calls for a systems approach in health care and in health sciences research that could evaluate multiple variables interacting in dynamic ways. As several panelists, including Dr. Lawrence Green, noted, this is a significant shortcoming of randomized trial methodology, which tests one variable at a time and is not designed to evaluate multifaceted preventive approaches, such as the lifestyle interventions described by Ornish. New, more appropriate assessment methods are under development. They range from improved effectiveness trials at the community level to studies of immune system biomarkers at the molecular level, to an array of study methods being used at the National Institutes of Health (NIH) National Center for Complementary and Alternative Medicine (NCCAM), described by Dr. Josephine Briggs.

Advances in genomic sciences are increasingly illuminating the contribution of genes to health and disease, explained Dr. Richard Lifton. New, more effective treatments may result that can be tailored to a person's genetic profile—a possibility that will greatly facilitate personalized medicine and person-centered care. However, as several panelists pointed out, "we are more than our genes," and it is the epigenetic influences—the interactions of genes with other factors—that shape health and illness. Dr. Mitchell Gaynor reported on numerous studies indicating the influence of diet and other environmental factors on the expression of genes and, consequently, their effects on health.

Psychosocial factors including stress, loneliness, and depression, all mediated by the brain, were described by McEwen and Dr. Esther Sternberg as strong contributors to health and disease. As the brain responds to stress, hormones are released that can, for example, interfere with the immune response and metabolic processes and damage the cardiovascular system. Something as simple as having a support group, a wide social network, or a nurturing belief system helps people manage stress and recover from illness, Ornish and Sternberg said. People with high levels of stress can be found throughout society. Dr. Nancy Adler noted that people in lower socioeconomic strata are particularly vulnerable to the effects of stress, which is reflected in their lower health status and premature aging at the cellular level.

Panelists said that lifestyle choices are important not only because unhealthy choices contribute to many of the leading causes of mortality, but also because healthy choices hold the potential to outperform commonly prescribed drugs, increase brain function, and affect the expression of genes. As individuals around the world begin to adopt an "American" lifestyle, especially our diet, the challenges of preventive medicine are becoming global, Ornish said.

SCIENCE KEYNOTE ADDRESS
Dean Ornish, Preventive Medicine Research Institute and University of California, San Francisco

The good physician treats the disease;
the great physician treats the patient
who has the disease.
—Sir William Osler

Ornish is a scientist and clinician who has spent much of the last three decades conducting clinical studies in what is now called integrative medicine. He described integrative medicine, or "prospective medi-

cine," as *predictive, preventive, personalized, and participatory* (Snyderman and Williams, 2003; Weston and Hood, 2004). While it provides
the best conventional care, its principal focus is on the preventive maintenance of health by attention to all components of lifestyle, including
diet, exercise, stress management, and emotional well-being. Lifestyle
choices offer many opportunities to improve health, as these decisions
are made multiple times throughout every day. Integrative medicine may
also be perceived as "functional medicine," which focuses on the underlying pathways of chronic disease, such as inflammation, genetics, and
metabolism (Bland, 2008; Hyman, 2007). Integrative medicine takes a
systems approach to improving patient health, and analyses of its effectiveness also must examine systemic, synergistic effects. Integrative
medicine contrasts with that of conventional medicine, where, Ornish
said, clinicians spend a great deal of time mopping up the floor around an
overflowing sink instead of just turning off the faucet.

Evidence in integrative medicine accumulates, not through studies
involving one independent variable and one dependent variable, but
rather through studies of the effects of multiple factors working together
in systematic ways. Similar to the components of a light bulb, the whole
is greater than the sum of the parts.

Ornish gave an example of the synergy of integrative medicine that
is demonstrated in a study of curcumin—a component of the spice tur-
meric, an ingredient in Indian curries. Curcumin, he noted, is known to
have anti-inflammatory and antitumor properties, suppressing the onco-
gene MDM2; further, as a free radical scavenger, it inhibits oxidative
DNA damage and may help prevent Alzheimer's disease. Researchers
have hypothesized that India's substantially lower incidence of Alzheimer's disease might be associated with curcumin ingestion because it
suppresses inflammation that, in turn, leads to amyloid deposits in the
brain that lead to Alzheimer's disease. Initial studies of curcumin alone
failed to show any beneficial effect. However, he reported, when it is
combined with black pepper, as it often is in local cuisine and in Ay-
urvedic medicine, there was about a 20-fold increase in curcumin's
bioavailability, demonstrating a synergistic effect of the spices (Shoba et
al., 1998).

Similarly, other studies show that a diet rich in fruit and vegetables
protects against heart disease and some forms of cancer, although vitamins alone usually do not. For example, foods containing beta-carotene
and other carotinoids have various health benefits, most likely owing to
their antioxidant effect. Yet, in some circumstances, beta-carotene die-

tary supplements appear to have a *pro*-oxidant effect and actually in-crease the risk of lung cancer among smokers. Smoking causes inflam-mation in the lungs, a condition that increases free radicals that can damage DNA. In a recent study, beta-carotene supplements were shown to further increase free radicals in a smoker's airways (van Helden et al., 2009). This increase occurs because supplemental beta-carotene inhibits an enzyme called myeloperoxidase and *increases* the formation of hy-droxyl free radicals, leading to increased inflammation and oxidative stress. Thus, dietary beta-carotene inhibits inflammation whereas sup-plements can increase it; studying beta-carotene in isolation (supple-ments) can miss the benefit of beta-carotene in foods and result in misleading information.

The third example Ornish gave of synergy in integrative medicine research was a 1989 study in which a group of women was treated with chemotherapy, radiation, and surgery for metastatic breast cancer. One study cohort, randomly assigned to a support group that met 1 hour a week, exhibited a 5-year survival rate twice as high as that of control subjects who did not participate in a support group (Spiegel et al., 1989). "If a new drug had been shown to do that, it would be malpractice not to prescribe it," Ornish said. However, more recent studies failed to repli-cate this result.

The possible explanation for this result came in 2007, in research re-porting that there was no *overall* survival in support group participants, but there *was* a survival advantage for women with estrogen receptor (ER)-negative breast cancer (Spiegel et al., 2007). Apparently, hormonal therapy improved so much after 1989 in ER-positive breast cancer (but not ER-negative breast cancer) that it washed out the contribution of support groups for those who were ER-positive, while the benefit of sup-port groups still occurs among ER-negative women. Among ER-negative women, those who participated in the support group still had survival rates 25 percent greater than those who did not (Spiegel et al., 2007). Without looking at the larger context—the system—this effect would have been missed.

Integrative Medicine and Pathways of Disease

Awareness, in Ornish's view, is the first step in healing. One prop-erty of science is its power to raise awareness. Science can help us un-derstand that what we do, how we feel, and what happens to us are all interconnected. Clinical research in various aspects of integrative medicine have produced dramatic evidence of the effects of lifestyle on health status and suggested the importance of taking a systems approach and considering factors other than those traditionally held responsible for causing not only chronic disorders but also infections diseases.

Health and disease are much more multidimensional than once thought—for example, not everyone who is infected with a virus gets sick. Psychosocial factors significantly affect this varying susceptibility. For example, HIV-positive patients who were depressed were twice as likely to develop AIDS, and to die of it, than were HIV-infected patients without depression (Burack et al., 1993; Mayne et al., 1996). Depression prompted a significantly more rapid health decline, measured by cell death and reduced lymphocyte counts. Similarly, volunteers infected with a rhinovirus were less likely to develop head colds if they had extensive social supports (Cohen et al., 1997). Subjects with at least six interpersonal relationships—manifested in phone calls or visits—were only one-fourth as likely to develop cold symptoms.

Reactions to stress are a well-recognized factor in immune function and can be either health protecting or health damaging. Stress generally suppresses immune function, while relaxation and meditation enhance it. Thus, there can be synergy between meditation and allopathic interventions. For example, psoriasis patients' skin cleared much faster (60 percent after 50 days) if they received standard photochemotherapy *and* listened to mindfulness-based stress management tapes; lesions of patients who did not use the tapes were only 20 percent clear after 50 days (Bernhard et al., 1988).

Integrative Medicine and Lifestyle Change

Many people mistakenly believe that only a new drug or a new and expensive technology can succeed against disease. Ornish and his team use high-tech, state-of-the-art measurement techniques to show the benefits of low-tech, low-cost, and, in some cases, ancient interventions and forms of disease prevention. Comprehensive lifestyle changes—including changing what we eat, how we respond to stress, moderate exercise, and greater love and intimacy—can yield remarkable improvements in health. Equally as important, these improvements are experienced within a short timeframe, which helps individuals feel better and facilitates the sustainability of their lifestyle modifications.

Early in his career, Ornish conducted several studies to evaluate the effects of lifestyle on heart disease. In the first study, 10 heart disease patients who undertook comprehensive lifestyle changes for only 1 month experienced a 90 percent reduction in angina as well as improved blood flow (myocardial perfusion) to their hearts, the first study showing that coronary heart disease may be reversed by changing lifestyle (Ornish et al., 1979). In the second study, a randomized controlled trial, a similar set of patients experienced a 91 percent reduction in angina and a significant increase in the heart's ability to pump blood, while the control group experienced a decrease (Ornish et al., 1983). In later randomized trials, patients who made comprehensive lifestyle changes showed a significant reduction in coronary artery blockages (atherosclerosis) as measured by quantitative coronary arteriography after 1 year and an even greater reversal of heart disease after 5 years, whereas the randomized control group showed a worsening of coronary atherosclerosis after 1 year (Ornish et al., 1990) and greater worsening after 5 years (Ornish et al., 1998), as shown in Figure 4-1. Cardiac PET scans revealed that 99 percent of patients who made these lifestyle changes were able to stop or reverse the progression of their heart disease (Gould et al., 1995).

In a subsequent study, comprehensive lifestyle changes appeared to significantly slow, stop, or reverse the progression of early-stage prostate cancer, the first time that an integrative medicine intervention was shown to affect the progression of any form of cancer in a randomized controlled trial (Ornish et al., 2005). In both the cardiac and prostate cancer studies, the more people changed their lifestyle, the more benefit they received in a dose–response effect. If borne out, this finding is empowering, as the degree of improvement may be more a function of adherence than age or disease severity.

Lifestyle changes can even outperform drugs in the secondary prevention of disease. In diabetes, lifestyle modifications functioned better than metformin in preventing the adverse effects of diabetes, including damage to the eyes, nerves, and kidneys (Knowler et al., 2002). One's own body, Ornish suggested, may be able to regulate blood sugar levels more consistently than drugs, in these conditions.

The idea that taking a pill is easy but changing lifestyle is difficult, if not impossible, is not supported by the evidence, said Ornish. Studies show that two-thirds of patients prescribed statin drugs are not taking them only 4 months later because these drugs do not make people feel

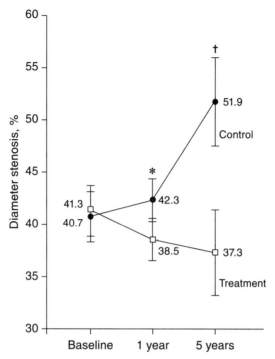

FIGURE 4-1 Mean percentage diameter stenosis in treatment and control groups at baseline, 1 year, and 5 years.
NOTES: Mean percentage diameter stenosis in treatment and control groups at baseline, 1 year, and 5 years. Error bars represent SEM; asterisk, $P = .02$ by between-group 2-tailed test; dagger, $P = .001$ by between-group 2-tailed test.
SOURCE: Ornish et al., 1998. Reproduced from *JAMA* 280(23):2001-2007 (December 16, 1998), with permission. Copyright 1998 American Medical Association. All rights reserved.

better (Ornish, 2009). In contrast, Ornish said that comprehensive lifestyle changes are dynamic, and often cause people to feel so much better, so quickly, that it reframes the reason for changing lifestyle from risk factor reduction (which is boring) or fear of dying (which is too frightening) to joy of living.

Ornish noted that moderate changes in lifestyle create only moderate benefits. For example, people who are diagnosed with hypercholesterolemia are often asked to make moderate changes in diet, but these relatively small changes cause negligible reductions in LDL cholesterol. Conversely, those who made more intensive changes in diet and lifestyle experienced a 40 percent average reduction in LDL cholesterol, comparable to what can be achieved with statin drugs without the costs ($18 billion for Lipitor last year) and potential side effects (e.g., muscle and liver damage) (Ornish et al., 1998).

Effects of Lifestyle Changes on Brain Function and Gene Expression

Ornish provided several examples of how lifestyle changes can improve brain function. Evidence exists that healthy diets, effective management of stress, moderate exercise, and being in loving relationships can produce growth in neurons, through the newly appreciated phenomenon of neuroplasticity. Consuming such foods as chocolate, blueberries, and tea, as well as alcohol in moderate amounts, can cause neurogenesis, whereas saturated fats, sugar, nicotine, and excessive consumption of alcohol can speed up the death of brain cells. Interestingly, he said, cannabinoids may increase neurogenesis, but opiates and cocaine decrease it. Depression and chronic feelings of stress reduce hippocampal volume and therefore impair memory (Campbell et al., 2004; Conrad, 2006; Sheline et al., 2003). In contrast, increased exercise has been associated with an increase in hippocampal volume within only a few months, as demonstrated in Figure 4-2 (Erickson and Kramer, 2009). Increases in brain size in the hippocampus and frontal cortex have been also associated with cognitive therapy, stress management, and psychotherapy (de Lange et al., 2008).

Changes in lifestyle affect gene expression—as nurture, in some cases, trumps nature. The Gene Expression Modulation by Intervention with Nutrition and Lifestyle (GEMINAL) studies found beneficial effects in 501 genes within 3 months after comprehensive lifestyle changes, including meditation. Changes in gene expression included the down-regulating of genes that promote heart disease or cancer and up-regulation of tumor-suppressing genes (Dusek et al., 2008; Ornish et al., 2008a). Ornish reiterated that genes are not destiny, and that genomics can be an important platform in studying the effects of integrative medicine.

Lifestyle change also has been shown to affect telomere length, which plays a role in aging and longevity. The effect of stress on telomere length was demonstrated in a study of women who felt highly stressed, as long-time caregivers of children with autism or birth defects.

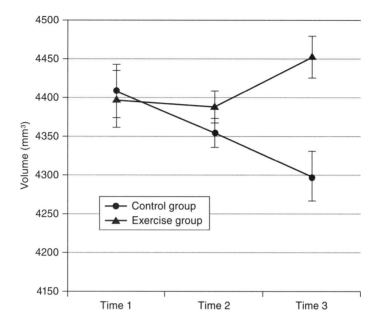

FIGURE 4-2 Hippocampus volume change.
SOURCE: Reproduced from *British Journal of Sports Medicine*, K.I. Erickson and A. F. Kramer, 43(1):22-24, 2009 with permission from BMJ Publishing Group Ltd.

These women exhibited lower levels of telomerase, the enzyme that repairs and lengthens damaged telomeres (Epel et al., 2004). The women's perception of stress was highly correlated with shorter telomeres. In contrast, comprehensive lifestyle changes led to almost 30 percent increases in telomerase, and thus telomere length, within 3 months, as shown in Figure 4-3 (Ornish et al., 2008b). Ornish commented that this was the first study showing that any intervention can increase telomerase, another example that integrative medicine interventions are not only as good as pharmaceutical interventions but often better, much less expensive, and that the only side effects are good ones.

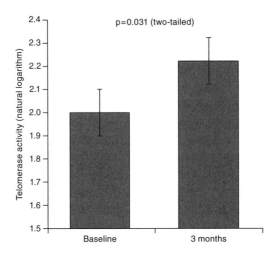

FIGURE 4-3 Increase in telomerase activity from baseline to 3 months.
SOURCE: Reprinted from *Lancet Oncology*, Vol. 9, Ornish, D., J. Lin, J. Daubenmier, G. Weidner, E. Epel, C. Kemp, M. J. Magbanua, R. Marlin, L. Yglecias, P. R. Carroll, and E. H. Blackburn, Increased telomerase activity and comprehensive lifestyle changes: A pilot study, Pages 1048-1057, Copyright 2008, with permission from Elsevier.

A globalization of chronic diseases such as heart disease, diabetes, and cancer is occurring, as other countries are starting to eat like us, live like us, and die like us—a trend that is almost completely preventable, said Ornish. Through lifestyle change, preventive medicine can reap benefits on a global scale. Ornish also pointed out that the choices we make in our personal lives affect our planet as well. For example, some suspect that more global warming is caused by livestock consumption (due to methane production) than from all forms of transportation combined.

Limitations of Conventional Medicine and Traditional Research

Diet and lifestyle changes that have already proved effective could prevent 95 percent of heart disease (Yusuf et al., 2004), Ornish said. However, a series of randomized controlled trials has shown that the usual course of treatment that consists of angioplasty and bypass surgery and costs the nation more than $100 billion annually—does not prevent heart attacks or prolong life for the great majority of patients who receive them (Boden et al., 2007). An evidence-based approach to health care is necessary, he said, and should be applied across the board to conventional and integrative interventions alike. Instead, the dominant approach tilts toward reimbursement-based medicine rather than evidence-based medicine.

Conventional methodologies available for gathering evidence on integrative medicine are often limited. Randomized controlled trials (RCTs) may work well for controlling bias in drug trials and are considered the gold standard for evaluating new treatments. However, lifestyle interventions and systems approaches often introduce uncontrollable sources of bias, making RCTs a less suitable evaluation method for complex lifestyle interventions. The randomization of participants can be challenging in lifestyle interventions. All participants must go through a series of baseline tests and agree to commit to make lifestyle changes if they are assigned to the experimental group. However, participants who are then randomized to the control group may become disappointed or even angry about the assignment, because they believe the intervention may have been beneficial to them, and they often drop out of the study as a result. Unlike a drug study, in which access to a new drug can be limited to experimental group participants, researchers cannot prevent the control group from making positive lifestyle changes on their own, which will confound the study's results.

The study of integrative medicine cannot easily be limited to the study of only one independent variable and one dependent variable, noted Ornish. For example, if the intervention consists of exercise, additional independent variables may be involved, such as increased social interaction with others who are exercising with the participant. Such interactions provide encouragement and support, and reinforce the individual's sense of meaning, self-efficacy, and purpose. People who begin to exercise regularly are also likely to improve their diets. These additional variables can complicate the interpretation of study results.

New research methods are being devised to better assess integrative medicine interventions. One alternative, developed by Marvin Zelen, consists of a randomized invitational design. In this approach, participants are assigned to a study group before being interviewed, so that the intervention is not described in detail to those assigned to the control group, and they do not have to commit to participate in the intervention before randomization. Members of the control group are asked only to agree to be tested; subsequently, they are less likely to drop out and tend not to be upset about the assignment. Crossover designs, in which the control group does not receive the intervention initially (and can serve as a nonintervention control group) but later receives the intervention, also can improve study design. Sham interventions are another approach that has been used in acupuncture studies. In this approach, members of the control group receive needle placements but not in the radial locations used in acupuncture (Haake et al., 2007). Innovative experimental designs and systems approaches such as these can lead to more persuasive evidence.

Transforming Human Experience

To Ornish, the most prevalent epidemic among Americans is not heart disease, cancer, or obesity, but rather loneliness and depression. Antidepressants are one of the nation's most frequently prescribed drugs. Study after study has shown that people who feel lonely and depressed are many times more likely to get sick and to die prematurely than people who have a sense of love, connection, and community, said Ornish. This effect is, in part, because lonely and depressed individuals are more likely to smoke, overeat, drink too much, and work too hard, but it also involves mechanisms that are not completely understood. For example, within 6 months after a heart attack, patients who were depressed were six times more likely to die than patients who were not—a finding that is independent of traditional risk factors, such as blood pressure and cholesterol levels, as shown in Figure 4-4 (Frasure-Smith et al., 1993). Animal studies show similar results: rabbits that were talked to, petted, played with, and essentially loved had 60 percent less plaque in their arteries than a group that was neglected (Nerem et al., 1980), even though these rabbits were genetically comparable and on the same diet.

In a final observation, Ornish described that sustainable changes in lifestyle are based on joy, fun, pleasure, and freedom, not austerity and deprivation. The language of behavioral change, unfortunately, often has a moralistic quality—or what he termed a fascist quality: "I cheated on my diet" and "I ate bad food, so I'm a bad person." Willpower and patient compliance are based on restricting and manipulating behavior, which is not sustainable. The mechanisms that respond to comprehensive lifestyle changes are much more dynamic than had once been realized,

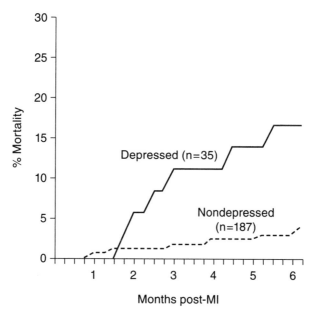

FIGURE 4-4 Cumulative mortality for depressed and nondepressed patients. NOTE: MI = myocardial infarction SOURCE: Frasure-Smith et al., 1993. Reproduced from *JAMA* 270(15):1819-1825 (October 20, 1993), with permission. Copyright 1998 American Medical Association. All rights reserved.

and, as described earlier, they allow patients to experience significant improvements in how they feel in a relatively short time. As Ornish described, "Joy of living is a more sustainable and powerful motivator than fear of dying. How *well* we live is more motivating than how *long* we live." Meditation, for example, was not used by spiritual teachers to unclog arteries or improve genes, but rather to help quiet minds and bodies in order to experience an inner sense of peace, joy, and well-being.

Ornish concluded by sharing an anecdote from a friend and teacher with whom he had studied, Swami Satchidananda. When asked the difference between wellness and illness, Satchidananda replied by writing the words on a blackboard and circling the *I* in illness and the *we* in wellness. Healing occurs when we move from the loneliness, isolation, and depression of the *I* toward the sense of support, connection, and community of the *we*.

PANEL ON THE SCIENCE BASE
FOR INTEGRATIVE MEDICINE

Panel Introduction
Bruce S. McEwen, The Rockefeller University

McEwen began the science panel with a brief summary of the biological effects of stress and the important role of the brain in mediating them. The brain is the central organ of stress; it perceives and decides what is threatening, producing physiologic responses that lead to adaptation and behavior that promotes or damages health, as shown in Figure 4-5. Although the body has a formidable capacity to defend itself against stress, this capacity is compromised by allostatic load—the cumulative, damaging effects of the overuse or disregulation of stress response systems over time—that results from chronic stress and behavior associated with experiencing stress, such as overeating, poor sleep, and lack of physical activity.

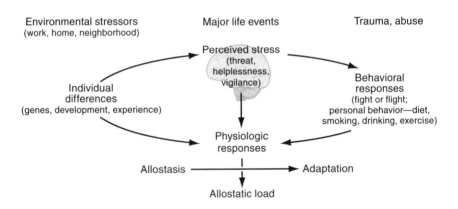

FIGURE 4-5 The stress response and development of allostatic load.
NOTES: The perception of stress is influenced by one's experiences, genetics, and behavior. When the brain perceives an experience as stressful, physiologic and behavioral responses are initiated, leading to allostasis and adaptation. Over time, allostatic load can accumulate, and the overexposure to mediators of neural, endocrine, and immune stress can have adverse effects on various organ systems, leading to disease.
SOURCE: McEwen, 1998. Reprinted, with permission, from *New England Journal of Medicine.* Copyright 1998 by Massachusetts Medical Society.

Stress mediators, such as adrenalin and cortisol, are a part of a complex nonlinear network in which mediators regulate each other. These mediation pathways include parasympathetic as well as sympathetic activity. Other players in the network are oxidative stress, which is essential for life but when excessive has deleterious effects, and anti-inflammatory and inflammatory cytokines, which are highly important in the adaptation of the immune system. These important mediators and others concurrently affect brain and metabolic functions, as well as the cardiovascular and immune systems, sometimes producing comorbidities.

In considering the science of integrative medicine, McEwen emphasized the lasting effects of early-life adversity and stress. As the CDC Adverse Childhood Experiences studies and others have shown, low socioeconomic status can lead to problems in systemic pathophysiology as well as poor cognitive abilities and learning skills. Abuse, neglect, and chaos at home can result in a sense of helplessness, low self-esteem, distress, and poor self-regulatory behaviors. All of these stressors can cause early-life obesity, blood pressure elevation, cardiovascular reactivity, lasting inflammation, mental health problems, and, ultimately, a shorter life span (Lantz et al., 1998; Mare, 1990; Pamuk et al., 1998; Pappas et al., 1993). Family stressors are found not only among people of low socioeconomic status, but span all socioeconomic strata and have many physical and mental health consequences for the children and adults (Repetti et al., 2002).

McEwen noted that the panel was organized to begin broadly with social determinants of health and progress through to genetics, epigenetics, and research methods. Advancing scientific methods have provided rapidly expanding data on gene expression and patterns of inheritance. Yet, as several other speakers indicated, the social environment exerts a powerful influence on health.

Social Determinants of Health
Nancy E. Adler, University of California, San Francisco

Dr. Nancy Adler offered the perspective that, even though many types of risk occur in all socioeconomic groups, the ability to make lifestyle changes and to engage in healthy lifestyles is often patterned by social status. She reminded the summit participants that the people most in need of the integrative medical interventions being discussed are frequently the people least able to access them, due to social barriers.

Socioeconomic status (SES) typically includes the triad of income, education, and occupation. The higher one is positioned on any of these three ladders, the better one's health status is likely to be. More than 3 in 10 adults living below the federal poverty level[1] rate their health as fair or poor, whereas less than 7 percent of adults in the highest income group rate their health fair or poor (Robert Wood Johnson Foundation, 2008). This effect is most prominent in the health status gap between people below the poverty level compared to those just above it, as indicated in Figure 4-6a. Every study of the relationship between health and income confirms that health status is directly related to income.

Education shows similar results, as seen in Figure 4-6b. There is a four- to five-fold health difference in reported fair or poor health between college graduates and those with less than a high school diploma, with improved health among people at each step of additional education (Robert Wood Johnson Foundation, 2008). Although income may be affected by reverse causation—poor health can cause a drop in income—education is relatively free of this effect.

Children exhibit the same general pattern, when socioeconomic status is measured in terms of their parents' income and education, as shown in Figures 4-7a and 4-7b. Fortunately, children generally are much healthier than adults, so the percentages of children in poor health are smaller.

One way to conceptualize the effect of socioeconomic status (SES) on health is that lower SES accelerates the aging process by increasing allostatic load, as discussed by McEwen. People who are disadvantaged experience the physical changes of aging earlier in life, including higher blood pressure, higher body mass index, greater abdominal fat deposition, and shallower evening drop in cortisol, said Adler.

The powerful relationship between health and SES is apparent even at the level of cellular aging, as reflected in telomere length. One illustration of this involves the third component of SES, occupation. English

---

[1]Each year, the Department of Health and Human Services publishes the Federal Poverty Income Guidelines in the *Federal Register*. These guidelines are often referred to as the "federal poverty level," and they provide the total annual income level at which families of various sizes are considered impoverished.

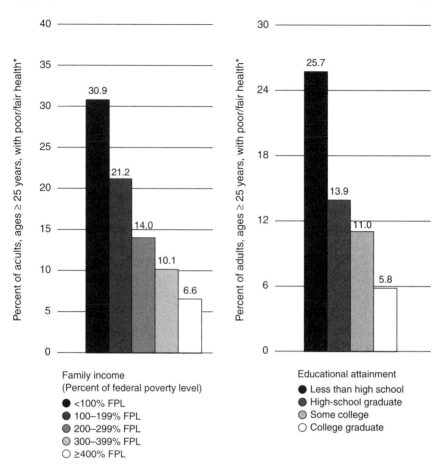

FIGURE 4-6a and 4-6b Relationship between income and education and reported adult health status.

NOTE:*age-adjusted.

SOURCE: Robert Wood Johnson Foundation, 2008. Reprinted, with permission. Copyright 2008 Robert Wood Johnson Foundation/Overcoming Obstacles to Health. Prepared by the Center on Social Disparities in Health at the University of California, San Francisco; and Norman Johnson, U.S. Bureau of the Census, using data from the National Longitudinal Mortality Study, 1988–1998.

workers in manual occupations showed a decrease of 140 base pairs in telomeres when compared to same-age workers in nonmanual fields, as shown in Figure 4-8; this is comparable to 8 years of aging (Cherkas et al., 2006).

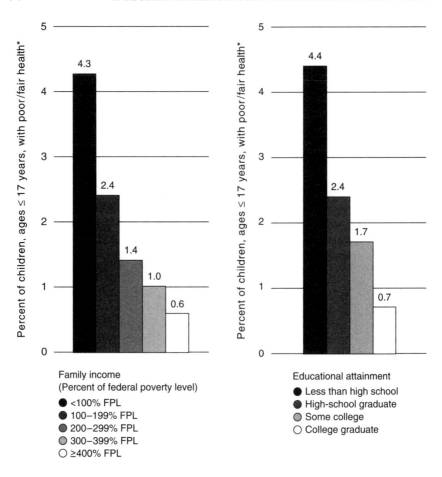

FIGURE 4-7a and 4-7b Relationship between income and education and reported child health status.

NOTE: *age-adjusted.

SOURCE: Robert Wood Johnson Foundation, 2008. Reprinted with permission. Copyright 2008 Robert Wood Johnson Foundation/Overcoming Obstacles to Health. Prepared by the Center on Social Disparities in Health at the University of California, San Francisco. Source: National Health Interview Survey, 2001–2005.

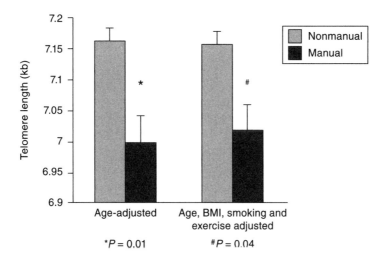

FIGURE 4-8 Mean telomere length and standard error by manual vs. non-manual social class groupings.
SOURCE: Cherkas et al., 2006. Reprinted, with permission, from *Aging Cell*, 2006. Copyright 2006 The Authors.

SES shapes almost every aspect of people's lives. It affects where they work, where they live, the social norms that govern them, where their children are educated, and their physical and social environments. In turn, these environments affect more proximal causes of disease and health, such as health behavior, access to health care, and exposure to toxins and pathogens, as well as to social threats that generate stress responses.

The current model of health focuses on the individual, involving efforts to promote behavior change, reduce stress, and increase patient empowerment. However, to improve health, it may be more effective to attempt broader strategies, suggested Adler. For example, Kaiser Permanente in the San Francisco Bay area responded to low-income individuals' lack of access to fresh fruits and vegetables by sponsoring farmers' markets at its health facilities.

Environmental, social, economic, and educational policy and interventions can affect people's health-related behavior and their heath status; these can occur at the national and/or local level. The state of the science now adequately documents the effects of social factors in health.

The next challenge, Adler said, is to determine how best to use a comprehensive set of tools, ranging from policy change to clinical interventions, to make a difference in improving health.

Mind–Body Medicine
Esther M. Sternberg, National Institute of Mental Health

Biologic pathways mediated by the brain provide the central connection between the external environmental factors described by Adler and health status. Sternberg described these pathways, particularly those related to the immune response to stress. A stressor triggers a cascade of neuroendocrine activity. The hypothalamus and the pituitary gland produce the stress hormones CRH and ACTH, and, in response, the adrenal glands release cortisol—the body's most potent anti-inflammatory hormone. Cortisol also is vital in regulating the immune system by providing an opportunity for it to return to homeostasis after a stress event occurs. Concurrently, the adrenergic sympathetic nervous system releases norepinephrine, and the adrenal medulla produces adrenalin. Together, these nerve chemicals and hormones, regulate the immune response at the cellular and molecular levels.

Health requires effective communication between the neuroendocrine and immune systems. An imbalance between these systems can cause disease. Too much cortisol, for example, can increase susceptibility to infections. People with excess cortisol may have more frequent or severe viral infections, less benefit from vaccines, prolonged wound healing, increased vascularization of solid tumors, and increased chromosomal aging (Armaiz-Pena et al., 2009; Cohen et al., 2007; Kiecolt-Glaser et al., 1995). By contrast, people with a cortisol deficiency will have a diminished anti-inflammatory effect and increased susceptibility to such autoimmune inflammatory diseases as inflammatory arthritis. Research indicates that the development of cardiovascular disease, diabetes, and depression can be influenced by cortisol-related inflammation.

The road to healing also is modulated by the brain. Health-promoting activities, such as meditation, yoga, tai chi, and exercise, have biologic effects on the neuroendocrine systems. When people engage in these types of activities, the vagus nerve functions as a brake on the sympathetic nervous system, thereby increasing the power of certain components of the immune system. Also, such activities prompt release of powerful neuroendocrine system hormones (specifically, endorphins and dopamine).

There is now broad acceptance that stress and allostatic load, or cumulative effects of stress, can foster disease. However, less is known about how health and healing are affected by a person's beliefs—feelings of purpose, peace, relaxation—which are enhanced by meditation, yoga, mild to moderate exercise, and several other activities. The biology of belief is difficult to study in humans and impossible in animals. However, elegantly designed studies are beginning to shed light on brain mechanisms underlying such interventions. These include activation of the brain's positive emotional centers, with release of dopamine and endogenous opiates, and activation of the vagus nerve and parasympathetic nervous system, with resulting down-shifting of the stress response.

Sternberg conceded that she had been a skeptic of the relationship between belief and healing until she experienced inflammatory arthritis—an illness related to chronic stress—after caring for her terminally ill mother. She began to be convinced of the relationship while on holiday in Crete, when a routine of swimming and meditation at the ruins of the temple of Aesclepius, the Greek god of medicine and healing, provided a beginning for her healing process. Sternberg reiterated Ornish's point about the importance of allowing the body to heal itself, which often requires lifestyle change.

Researchers need complex measures to understand how, biologically, a whole host of molecules work together in response to stress, relaxation, and other factors Sternberg referred to as *belief*. Ideally, these measures should provide a molecular signature of health or disease for a specific person, around which tailored advice can be developed. Researchers at the NIH have developed a way to obtain reliable measures of several of the immune biomarkers of stress through having people wear a sweat patch for 24 hours. Analysis of the sweat avoids having to draw blood, a process that, naturally, creates the stress that researchers are trying to measure. These biomarkers are evaluated through sophisticated methodologies that use immunoaffinity chromatography and various types of sophisticated mass spectrometry analyses.

In one such study, sweat patch analysis showed that asymptomatic women with a history of depression had elevated levels of proinflammatory cytokines and NPY, an adrenalin-like nerve chemical (Cizza et al., 2008). These women also exhibited a reduction in vasoactive intestinal peptide, a marker of the parasympathetic vagus nervous system. This signature indicated that their stress response had shifted away from vagally mediated relaxation toward a sympathetic adrenalin-mediated response. The significance of this finding is its suggestion that, although these women were asymptomatic, biological remnants of their depression remained.

Such advanced research techniques will enable development of a full picture of the brain's hormone-production activities that both contribute to disease and promote wellness.

Genomic and Predictive Medicine
Richard P. Lifton, Yale University School of Medicine

Dr. Richard Lifton emphasized the role of basic science in understanding, preventing, and treating disease. Examples of integrative approaches to understanding and eliminating disease can be found in the development of prevention and treatment strategies for infectious diseases. These diseases profoundly affected the course of public health history and the lives of millions. Even our presidents have not remained untouched: Franklin Roosevelt contracted poliomyelitis, and Abraham Lincoln's son, Willie, died in the White House of typhoid fever. Malaria was once endemic in the Foggy Bottom area of Washington, DC, where the summit was held. Many of these diseases were eradicated through integrative approaches that began with basic science, including the development of vaccines for prevention, targeted therapies for specific infections, and improvements in public health and sanitation.

The current status of genomic and predictive medicine reflects 150 years of progress in the basic sciences, starting with Gregor Mendel's 1865 recognition of genetic factors and Thomas Hunt Morgan's 1910 discovery that genes lie on chromosomes. Other milestones include the 1944 identification of DNA as the genetic material, the 1953 unveiling of the structure of DNA, the 1960 characterization of the genetic code, and the entire sequencing of the human genome in 2001. This last achievement allows the identification of all genes and common variations, and the stage is now set for understanding the inherited and acquired variations in genes and gene expression that contribute to the development of disease.

Basic science and genetics have been necessary for an improved understanding of the pathogenesis of cardiovascular disease, chronic myelogenous leukemia, and HIV, among others. This greater understanding has, in turn, led to new treatments. Highly effective statins were developed following the mapping of the cholesterol biosynthetic pathways, identification of a mutation in the LDL cholesterol receptor, and the recognition of a causal relationship between increased cholesterol levels and heart disease.

Recent advances in the treatment of chronic myelogenous leukemia build on a long history of basic science: in 1963, researchers identified a chromosomal anomaly related to the disease; in the 1970s, they found a specific chromosomal rearrangement; and in the 1980s, the specific gene mutation. The pharmaceutical industry and a passionate physician then developed and directed the clinical trials that established the capacity of a single drug to induce remission for most patients. Similarly, basic science led to the identification of HIV-1, the virus that causes AIDS. Diagnostic tests were developed, and a host of new drugs, including reverse transcriptase inhibitors, protease inhibitors, and integrase inhibitors, have transformed this rapidly fatal disease into a manageable chronic condition.

The sequencing of the human genome provides tremendous ability to characterize genes and identify their roles in human disease. A variety of study designs can be used to harness the knowledge resident in the genome, including the single-gene mutations that produce large effects and suggest therapeutic targets; acquired somatic mutations in cancer; and comprehensive measurement of gene expression in diseased and healthy tissues, in order to identify underlying disease pathways. Additionally, scientists increasingly can resequence large portions of the genome, which will soon enable identification of important mutations.

Lifton illustrated the impact of these genomic techniques with examples of newly understood pathogenesis of certain diseases. In Alzheimer's disease, for example, rare mutations produce common lipoprotein variations that are major contributors to disease progression. Discoveries of inherited and acquired mutations of BRCA1 and BRCA2 genes have fundamentally changed the understanding of breast cancer. Within just the last year, mutations in the IDH1 gene have been identified that appear to be essential to the formation of glioblastoma multiforme in the brains of young patients. These advances allude to the tremendous promise of efforts to define the biology that connects genes to disease.

Such discoveries also can help ameliorate racial and ethnic disparities in disease prevalence and health outcomes, said Lifton. Examples include newly acquired knowledge about the role of common variants of MYH9 in causing kidney failure for African Americans with hypertension or HIV, and the role of common variants of PLPLA3 in increasing the risk of nonalcohol-related fatty liver disease in Hispanic Americans.

The path from gene identification to therapy is difficult and unpredictable. To further advance the science base for integrative medicine, Lifton perceived a need for at least five resources: (1) a robust scientific enterprise, where investigators with subject-matter expertise proceed from gene discovery to finding plausible points for therapeutic intervention; (2) far broader interactions between academia, where the scientific strength in biology resides, and the pharmaceutical industry, where talent in medicinal chemistry prevails; (3) enterprising ways to manage conflicts of interest; (4) well-designed clinical trials to define best practices; and (5) improved delivery systems to ensure that the public ultimately benefits from this substantial investment in science.

Lifton offered two complementary visions of the future. In one, patients are treated with drugs targeted to individual abnormalities, based on their genomic data. That will likely be the case for disorders in which differences among patients are large, such as in certain cancers. In the other vision, disease pathways and key nodes along those pathways will be identified, allowing for the development of population-based interventions. Examples of the latter approach could be used to address both behavioral and environmental factors, such as reducing salt intake in order to control blood pressure and reducing cholesterol levels in order to prevent heart disease. Lifton said that realizing both visions require a fundamental, science-based understanding of the causes of disease.

Environmental Epigenetics
Mitchell L. Gaynor, Weill-Cornell Medical Center
and Gaynor Integrative Oncology

Gaynor introduced the discussion of environmental epigenetics by noting that one in three Americans, at some point in his or her life, is going to hear the words, "You have cancer." The question at hand is to what extent one's chances of acquiring cancer or other diseases are the result of one's genetic endowment or other, more controllable factors? The answer is a combination of the two—while the genes one is born with cannot be controlled, how those genes are expressed can be. Gaynor illustrated this point by describing nutritional genomic and toxicogenomic studies that use mouse models. In these studies, toxicogenomics examines how various toxins can increase tumor-promoter genes and decrease tumor-suppressor genes. Conversely, nutritional genomics uses nutrients to reduce cancer risk by increasing expression of tumor-suppressing genes.

Agouti mice are typically born with a pale yellow coat and an elevated risk of developing diabetes, obesity, and eventually, cancer. However, pregnant female agouti mice that are fed a methyl-rich mixture of nutrients including folic acid, B_{12}, choline, and betaine (found in beets) produced "pseudoagouti" offspring. These mice are born with brown coats and no elevated risk of obesity, diabetes, or cancer (Waterland and Jirtle, 2003). Researchers have found that the mother's diet during pregnancy changes gene expression in the offspring, a positive change that is transmitted to subsequent generations.

Researchers have obtained the same overall result after administering a different nutrient, the soy extract genistein (Dolinoy et al., 2006). While the earlier diet provided additional methyl groups enabling the DNA methylation that caused the change in gene expression, the genistein affected histone formation, which also facilitated the methylation process.

Endocrine disruptors exist in plastic products, cosmetics, and pesticides and are stored in the body for decades. When pregnant mice were exposed to either of two endocrine disruptors, vinclozolin (a fungicide used on grapes and other fruits) and methoxychlor (a pesticide now used instead of DDT), 90 percent of their male offspring had a 70 percent decrease in sperm cells. This defect in the epigenome was inherited through four generations (Reik et al., 2001). It may be no coincidence that 11 percent of Americans have problems with fertility, Gaynor said.

Bisphenol A (BPA) is another possible example. Agouti mice that were exposed to BPA and then fed either genistein or a diet rich in methyl groups produced pseudoagouti offspring. The nutritional supplement protected these mice from the BPA-induced heritable changes (Dolinoy et al., 2007).

The incidence of breast cancer in American women has tripled, from one in 22 in 1960, to one in eight today. A geneticist at the University of Washington has found that women born with the BRCA1 or BRCA2 mutation before 1940 had a 24 percent risk of breast cancer, whereas such women born after 1940, as endocrine disruptors have become more prevalent in the environment, have a 67 percent risk. Simultaneously, the risk of ovarian cancer doubled for BRCA1 carriers, and increased 23 percent for BRCA2 carriers (King et al., 2003). These large increases in cancer risk suggest a significant gene–environment interaction, said Gaynor.

Women in societies that consume a great deal of soy, such as Japan, have one-seventh the incidence of fatal breast cancer as American women. Asian men living in Asian countries have one-thirtieth the incidence of fatal prostate cancers as American men. Gaynor suggested a close relationship between environmental public policy and personalized medicine, saying that often "The environment outside us is the same as the environment inside us."

Intervention Evaluation and Outcomes Measures
Lawrence W. Green, University of California, San Francisco

Green indicated that he approaches integrative medicine from the opposite end of the biopsychosocial spectrum than the previous panelists. Namely, he approaches it from the standpoint of public health. He noted progress has been made in public health since the development of the disease prevention and health promotion initiative in the late 1970s under Surgeon General Julius B. Richmond, Dr. Michael McGinnis, and others. Drawing from this experience, he contended that, in order to achieve more evidence-based practice, we need more practice-based evidence.

Patient-centered medicine, which is a hallmark of integrative care, challenges the supremacy of RCTs in evidence-based medicine, said Green. This challenge was acknowledged in 1999 in the preface to the second edition of a book by Archie L. Cochrane, whose previous contributions earned him the sobriquet of "father of evidence-based medicine," and it appropriately may be termed the "post-Cochrane challenge" (Cochrane, 1999).

A Venn diagram illustrates this challenge, as shown in Figure 4-9. There is a large circle of information (labeled C) that is potentially useful to patients in their decision making. This sphere overlaps a smaller sphere (B) of information that is potentially evidence based. The overlap is small, consisting of information that is both potentially useful to patients and potentially evidence based. Only a tiny sector of this overlap contains information already grounded in good evidence (labeled A), usually resulting from RCTs. Ten years after Cochrane offered this construct, researchers are finally recognizing the need to apply alternative designs and to develop new study designs to obtain a large body of evidence that will also be useful to patients, said Green. Difficult to undertake, and tethered to conditions that may be far removed from patients' true circumstances and desires, RCTs provide information of only limited value or utility for prevention.

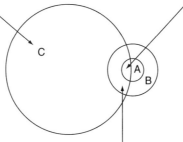

Information of importance to patient choice which is not even potentially of evidence-based type, e.g., information about the process of delivery of health care

Area where there is currently good evidence-based information which is of importance to patients in making choices

C

A

B

Information of importance to patient choice which is potentially of evidence-based type

A. Information which is currently based on good evidence
B. Information for which good-quality evidence-based information could be available in due course
C. Information which is potentially of importance to patients in making health care choices

FIGURE 4-9 Evidence-based medicine and integrative, patient-centered medicine.
SOURCE: Hope, T. 1997. Evidence-based patient choice and the doctor-patient relationship. In *But will it work, doctor?* London: Kings Fund. Reprinted, with permission from Tony Hope, The Ethox Center.

Research in integrative and person-centered medicine can shift the spotlight from the *mediating* variables that focus on the mechanisms of change to the *moderating* variables that focus on the characteristics of individual people and the context in which they live. Moderating variables are reflected in the types of questions a clinician asks patients in order to learn about their identity, values, lifestyle, and life conditions.

Green offered two strategic suggestions for meeting the post-Cochrane challenge. The first is to shape interventions in clinical research around moderating variables. Second, he emphasized the value of strategically blending theory and practical experience with evidence. An obsessive emphasis on best evidence has tended to crowd out good observational and theoretical considerations, he said. Theory permits us to generalize evidence to other populations, settings, and circumstances. This is especially useful when, as is almost always the case, replication of evidence may be too cumbersome, Green noted. Theory can help provide solutions to problems, so long as investigators draw on theories eclectically and do not start with a theory and then look for problems on which to test it. In the aphorism of computer scientist Jan van de Snepscheut, "Theory and practice are the same thing in theory, but they are not the same thing in practice." The same could be said of best evidence and practice.

Modalities in Complementary and Alternative Medicine
Josephine P. Briggs, National Center for
Complementary and Alternative Medicine

Briggs expressed the National Center for Complementary and Alternative Medicine's (NCCAM) commitment to integrative health care. NCCAM's mission is to build the evidence base for complementary and alternative medicine interventions. The NIH core principles that govern this mission include rigorous peer review, investigator-initiated science, and partnerships. NCCAM's annual budget of approximately $122 million constitutes only about 4.1 percent of all NIH expenditures. However, she reported that the center's programs generate a significant share of interest and excitement. All of NCCAM's large programs are operated through partnerships; partners include other NIH institutes and centers, other federal agencies, such as the Agency for Healthcare Research and Quality (AHRQ), and private-sector organizations.

The programs occupy four spheres: basic science, translational research, efficacy studies, and effectiveness research, as shown in Figure 4-10. Basic science consumes roughly half of NCCAM's resources. Current investigations in this area are evaluating the neuroscience of meditation, the biology of the placebo effect or expectancy effect, the neurobiological correlates of acupuncture, and neuroplasticity. An NCCAM-funded study in neuroplasticity, for example, demonstrated that a stroke patient imagining moving an arm affected by stroke increased movement and function in the affected arm. This may support the hypothesis that mental practice helps build neurocircuits for moving that arm (Page et al., 2007).

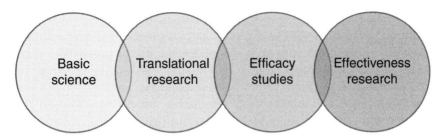

FIGURE 4-10 NCCAM's mission: Building the evidence base for integrative medicine.

Other basic science research includes investigation of natural foods and other natural products; epigenetics, including effects of stress on gene expression; and the role of prebiotics and probiotics in health. Although the basic science portfolio is thriving, NCCAM's limited funding means that these studies have the lowest grant application funding rates.

Efficacy studies make up about 12 percent of NCCAM's budget, including its signature RCTs of natural products and dietary supplements. For example, these investigations so far have found: no impact of *Echinacea* on the severity or frequency of head colds; positive substantial impacts of fish oil and omega-3 fatty acids on cardiovascular risk factors; and mostly negative results for ginkgo biloba, glucosamine and chondroitin, and St.-John's-wort. The results of these studies tend to affect consumer use of the products; for example, St.-John's-wort, which was widely used in 2002, is no longer among the top 20 nonvitamin, nonmineral, natural products used by adults, as reported by the 2007 National Health Interview Survey. Sometimes these types of studies lead to additional research. Further analysis of St.-John's-wort revealed that the active ingredient hypericin may not be the only active ingredient, as was initially expected. It is now thought that hyperforin, another compound in St.-John's-wort, may also be an important active ingredient.

Improved methodologies will be needed to evaluate complex complementary and alternative interventions in real-world settings. Effectiveness research, which is an expanding area of activity for NCCAM, is particularly ripe for new study designs. For example, use of sham interventions in acupuncture studies may describe certain effects but fails to show whether acupuncture is more effective than standard care.

Despite some assertions to the contrary, rigorous scientific studies can substantiate practices used in complementary and alternative medicine. To illustrate, in the management of chronic lower back pain, a peer-reviewed study supports the use of yoga (Sherman et al., 2005), a systematic (or Cochrane-type) review supports the use of manipulative exercise (Slade and Keating, 2007), and an authoritative clinical guideline includes recommendations to consider acupuncture, massage, spinal manipulation, and yoga among other approaches for patients who do not improve with self-care options (Chou and Huffman, 2007).

Now in its 10th year, NCCAM is embarking on a strategic planning process. Briggs solicited input from stakeholders and summit participants in this endeavor.

Panel Discussion

Members of the panel responded to questions from audience members in a discussion that was moderated by McEwen. Selected points of discussion follow.

Socioeconomic Status, the Environment, and Research

In response to a question on how research on integrative medicine can better involve lower-socioeconomic status (SES) populations, Adler observed that one attribute of low-SES groups is that they tend not to be well organized. Greater involvement of these patients may require going to where they are, through community-based research. Green agreed and noted that the NIH, Centers for Disease Control and Prevention (CDC), and the AHRQ are all supporting community-based participatory research. Green noted that one disadvantage of this approach is the need for an investigator to spend adequate time building trust in the community, but an advantage is that the community can help frame high-value research questions. An audience member took issue with the notion that minority populations are reluctant to participate in research projects; his organization's research has shown that the main factor in nonparticipation is that people were simply not asked to do so.

Several panelists responded to a related question regarding the lack of research on the effects of environmental risk factors and toxins on low-SES communities, where risks are often prevalent. Gaynor observed that African American women face an increased incidence of breast cancer as a result of increased exposure to endocrine-disrupting chemicals, which are found in many hair care products and cosmetics. He called for studying the relationships between endocrine disruptors and not only cancer, but also diabetes and obesity. Adler added that this point ties in with community-based research, as members of focus groups composed of inner-city residents have expressed concern about the health effects of toxins, dumpsites, and other local environmental hazards. Lifton noted that measuring the environment can be difficult. However, advances in measuring environmental effects on the body through evaluation of gene expression can be useful in recognizing harmful environmental agents. Sternberg suggested that proteomics can also be useful in analyzing biological changes that result from exposures.

Balancing High-Tech Interventions with Lifestyle and Environmental Changes

Panel members responded to the question of how to balance high-tech medical interventions and diagnostics with the broader impact of lifestyle and environmental health changes. Sternberg said that technology should be used as an advantage in advancing integrative medicine. She noted that high-tech methods can be used to assess the effects and health outcomes of lifestyle changes. Adler commented that skyrocketing health care costs create incentives to seek relatively inexpensive, low-tech interventions. Lifton mentioned the possibility of greater investment in disease prevention strategies, such as through changes in Medicare reimbursement.

Shifting the Paradigm

Panelists were asked to discuss how alternatives to RCTs could be developed. Green cited growing interest in this topic, as a result of the recent economic stimulus legislation, which contained support for comparative effectiveness research. He mentioned that large clinical trials often produce weak results; in the early 1980s, for example, the Multiple Risk Factor Intervention Trials ("MR. FIT"), a multi-intervention RCT, sought to reduce coronary heart disease in high-risk men. When no statistical difference in coronary deaths was found between the experimental and control groups, researchers sought to undertake subgroup analyses. Biostatisticians objected to analyzing the subgroups because they were not randomized, and subgroup analysis fell immediately into disrepute. Green suggested that subgroup analysis nevertheless offers the greatest potential to understand variations in moderating variables.

Briggs agreed with Green, indicating that RCT methods, developed in order to determine the efficacy of drugs, may not be sufficient to examine other types of interventions. Nor are they suited to assess the effectiveness of interventions in the real world, given all of the forms of heterogeneity in the U.S. population. Green urged that the different disciplines along the biopsychosocial spectrum resist the centrifugal force that pulls them into silos, and instead develop more transdisciplinary research approaches.

Gaynor commented that, in matters of protecting public health, the threshold for public policy interventions should be the precautionary principle, rather than 100 percent proof of effectiveness. The last half century could have been better spent in a war on carcinogenesis than in the war on cancer, he suggested. For example, much time was lost in accepting the tobacco industry's persistent claim that cigarettes were not proven to cause cancer. Adler added that a market model is lacking for making disease prevention profitable, and a better alignment of incentives is needed.

PRIORITY ASSESSMENT GROUP REPORT[2]

Advancing the Science Base

Lifton provided the report for the priority assessment group on advancing the science base. This summary includes the priorities discussed and was presented by the assessment group to the plenary session for its discussion and consideration; these priorities do not represent a consensus or recommendations from the summit.

The assessment group began with a discussion of one challenge that had resonated throughout the summit—one of definitions. The group noted that a difference exists between *integrative medicine* and an *integrated system*. The former involves the care of individual patients, while

---

[2]See Chapter 1 for a description of the priority assessment groups. Participants of this assessment group included Bruce McEwen (moderator), Richard Lifton (rapporteur), Donald Abrams, Kenneth Brigham, Margaret Chesney, Gary Deng, Wayne Jonas, Lixing Lao, Patrick Mansky, Rustum Roy, and Alan Trachtenberg.

the latter extends from basic science discovery all the way through the mechanisms of delivery and organization of care and to broad public health interventions.

In building the evidence base for integrative medicine, a pivotal task is establishing causal vectors. Genetics and genomics, in particular, have the capacity to demonstrate causation; within the next 3 to 5 years, these disciplines may revolutionize the understanding of some of the fundamental causes of health and wellness. In advancing this area of science, one participant noted the importance of recognizing biological variations among individuals when it comes to assessing effectiveness research on interventions.

Certain areas of biomedicine are not yet accorded sufficient attention among researchers, despite their importance and prevalence in population health. Areas that the group identified as requiring additional research and understanding were fatigue, the link between beliefs and biology, and the science of achieving behavior change. Fatigue is very prevalent in chronically ill patients, but scientists have not yet developed an understanding of its biologic foundations, nor is there funding support for research in this area. One disease where fatigue has received considerable attention is breast cancer. Findings in the area of fatigue should also be extended to increase the understanding of the role it plays in other conditions and diseases.

An increased understanding of the link between beliefs and biology, as described by Sternberg and others throughout the summit, and the effects of belief on physiology and human health are fundamental areas that the group suggested warrant additional research.

Progress is also needed in the development of evidence-based interventions for effective behavior change. Behavior change is a key strategy for preventing a very large number of diseases, but strategies for accomplishing it lack a great deal of empirical evidence. Additional research is required to improve the understanding of the various components of behavior change, including the effects of motivation, group support, and education. During the discussion with the audience, participants offered additional insight into ways to advance the science of behavior change. One participant suggested research involving a qualitative perspective—that is, asking individuals about their experiences and what meaning they attribute to behavioral change—may be a promising line of inquiry. Another suggestion was to apply the stages-of-change model used in psychology, which adjusts interventions to the individual's progress along the continuum from precontemplation to action.

To advance the science base of integrative medicine, including the priority areas identified for additional research, the assessment group determined that the most important set of key actors is research funders, including the NIH and private foundations. The role of funders in research is vital to providing incentives for shifts in research approaches. The group also noted that, while the biomedical research workforce has a strong basis, it requires more training in integrative human biology, behavior, and physiology. This additional training would show researchers how their work can apply to individual patients. One audience member reiterated this point and noted the importance of exposing doctorate-level bioscience students to the physicians and patients who ultimately use and benefit from their research.

5

Workforce and Education

Enlarge the opportunity, and the person will
expand to fill it.
—Eli Ginzberg

Dame Carol M. Black delivered the keynote for the summit session on workforce and education. Black described drivers and barriers of change in the area of workforce development and discussed the importance of "worklessness," or unemployment, in undermining health. In the panel discussion, moderated by Dr. Elizabeth A. Goldblatt, the panelists elaborated on the implications of advances in integrative medicine for the education and training of the nation's health professionals and researchers and discussed strategies for changing curricula, including interdisciplinary approaches, team-based training, and expansion of core competencies in healthy living and wellness.

An often-mentioned point in this session, described by Black and other panelists, is the need to expand interdisciplinary and multidisciplinary education to promote effective teamwork. This is increasingly important, because most health care interventions now require coordination and teamwork, said Sir Cyril Chantler. Yet, health practitioners typically are educated and trained in professional silos, hindering their ability to quickly transition and adapt to a team environment. Interprofessional education should begin early, particularly for physicians, to reinforce shared values and overcome the culture that rewards individual accomplishment, said Dr. Adam Perlman.

Demonstration projects also would be useful in developing more effective educational models for integrative health practitioners. One type of project, suggested by Dr. Mary Jo Kreitzer, would incorporate community health centers into interdisciplinary education opportunities. Another would involve training nonphysicians to be primary care providers; Dr. Richard Cooper viewed this prospect as inevitable, because of the looming shortage of primary care physicians. The latter model might be an appropriate outgrowth of developing new competencies for nurse practitioners and others. A third type of project, advocated and pioneered by Dr. Victoria Maizes, organizes training programs built around core competencies in integrative health.

Regardless of professional and specialty mix, health care practitioners today are not able to overcome some of the most important factors in health and disease—the socioeconomic factors raised by Black, such as employment, education, and poverty. In many respects, Cooper said, poverty constitutes the greatest of all the challenges facing the health care system.

WORKFORCE AND EDUCATION KEYNOTE ADDRESS
Carol M. Black, Academy of Medical Royal Colleges

> *Even in the most affluent countries, people who are less*
> *well off have substantially shorter life expectancies and*
> *more illnesses than the rich.*
> —*Richard Wilkinson and Michael Marmot*

Black began her keynote address by observing that the challenges facing the American and British health systems are remarkably similar and reflect global forces. There are several drivers to change within the realm of health care, many of which were described by other presenters throughout the summit and many of which are globally applicable. These drivers include expectations of the public and of individual patients, inequalities in health and health care, variations in the quality of care, health needs reflecting demographic shifts, the impact of lifestyle on health, advances in medical sciences, rising costs, and inefficiencies and failings of the system, Black noted. These many drivers suggest a needed analysis of whether education is appropriately aligned to overcome important barriers to change and meet the needs of the population.

Person-Centered Care and the Social Determinants of Health

Expectations of the health care system begin with care that is safe, effective, easy to access, and of high quality. People also want care that is personal; they want it to be geared to their own understanding of health and their expectations for restored or maintained capacity. Person-centered care should provide direct advice and support on lifestyle choices, such as smoking, nutrition, exercise, and drugs and alcohol. It also should offer support and advocacy for family problems, poverty, housing, and education. Unfortunately, the health professions education systems are not focused on the personal aspects of care. Personal care is compromised by time pressures on clinicians; the average seven-minute patient encounter with British physicians is not conducive to developing a therapeutic relationship.

Truly person-centered care will take into account the socioeconomic determinants of health, which include poverty or wealth, stress, early life experiences, social support or exclusion, work and unemployment, addiction, nutrition, oral health, and transportation (Marmot, 2004). Combined, these factors are major influences on longevity and health status throughout the course of one's life, and they need to be considered in the development of health policy, said Black. This shift would entail providing incentives for promoting healthy ways of living, rather than primarily reimbursing drugs and surgery (Chopra et al., 2009).

Relationship of Work and Health

Employment is one of the leading modifiers of health and illness, yet it is a factor rarely recognized by the health care system. Work has long been recognized as a fundamental social determinant of health. Galen observed that employment is nature's physician and is essential to human happiness; Voltaire said it banished boredom and poverty; and Osler said it brings hope to the young, confidence to the middle-aged, and repose to the elderly. Theodore Roosevelt declared, "Far and away the best prize that life offers is the chance to work hard at work worth doing." The findings of nearly 500 articles about the positive effects of work on physical and mental health and well-being were recently compiled in a single review (Waddell and Burton, 2006).

The long-term effects of worklessness require special attention in the current recession, suggested Black. Worklessness—especially over a long term—is a greater risk to health than many diseases. It poses greater risks to health than many hazardous occupations, such as construction, and it doubles or triples the risk of mental illness. Children who grow up in workless families have a five times greater incidence of mental illness than children living in a family with stable employment. Illness related to worklessness and work absences related to sickness cost the United Kingdom £100 billion annually, the same as the cost of running the National Health Service.

Black noted that while health care providers often discuss many health behavior and environmental factors with their patients, they rarely discuss patients' employment in a meaningful way. Health care providers need to know about the benefits of good work; they should use return to functional capacity and to work as a clinical indicator of success; and they should be aware of work-related concerns in the health care setting, such as communication with employers. Efforts are now under way in the United Kingdom to develop training programs that help physicians, especially in family medicine, focus on the health aspects of work and worklessness.

Workforce Reorientation

Meeting the expectations of patients and the public, providing person-centered care, and incorporating greater awareness of social determinants of health into health care necessitates change in health professional education. Trust, the fundamental component in the relationship between patients and providers, requires providers who demonstrate a number of attributes that include communication skills, empathy, nonjudgmental behavior toward patients, integrity, a commitment to quality and safety, and the ability to work in teams. Black noted that these attributes should be instilled throughout the education process.

Teamwork is especially important in meeting public expectations and addressing social determinants of health. Teamwork within professions and across professions is an increasingly essential component of success in health care; it also helps solidify relationships with both patients and other providers. Effective teamwork includes the ability to transfer tasks within a multiprofessional team, especially as tasks traditionally performed by physicians devolve on other professionals in the care team. Teamwork also includes competence in the coordination of care, which requires awareness of the skills and attributes of other team members. Yet, teamwork is an area of weakness in physician education and training. In the United Kingdom, teamwork in health care has been found to be somewhat unstructured, short-lived, rushed, and opportunistic, rather than strategic.

To meet the need for change in workforce education, the Academy of Medical Royal Colleges in the United Kingdom has developed a Medical Leadership Competency Framework that encompasses five domains: personal qualities, working with others, managing services, improving services, and setting direction. Each of the five domains includes subdirectives. For example, working with others includes developing collaborative networks, building and maintaining relationships, and encouraging others to contribute, as is shown in Figure 5-1. The framework includes a generic curriculum for physician training that can be adjusted to specific specialties. Use of the framework in the training of nurses and dentists is also planned.

The competency framework highlights teamwork. Black emphasized that all health professions students should learn to collaborate effectively across disciplines, because the best health care plan may include a combination of treatments provided by diverse practitioners. Some health professionals may fear losing their professional identity within a team, but clustering in teams tends to be additive to professional skills and knowledge, as each team member provides unique expertise.

Specialty Distribution of Health Professionals and Medical Education

Changing educational content to focus on teamwork is only one way to meet rising public expectations and address patients' full needs, including those involving the social determinants of health. Another vital aspect of change involves shortages of practitioners in some fields, such as gaps arising from the unbalanced specialty distribution of physicians. Black noted that concern exists in both the United States and the United Kingdom that too many physician specialists, such as surgeons, and too few primary care physicians are being trained. Additionally, new cohorts of health professionals may be required to adequately meet the health needs of the populations in an integrated way. Nursing, Black said, has a seminal relationship to integrative medicine, and much of what is now called complementary and alternative medicine has sat within the domain of nursing for generations. Nurses are educated to be holistic practitioners—attentive to mind, body, and spirit, and with an understanding of

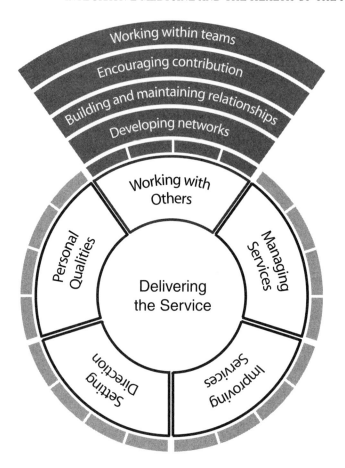

FIGURE 5-1 Competency framework: Working with others.
SOURCE: National Health Service Institute for Innovation and Improvement, 2009.

the range of complementary therapies that are available. To advance the workforce and redress imbalances, advances in medical education are necessary. Lifestyle and prevention need to be the cornerstones of the future health care system and thus a larger component of education.

To help produce the necessary changes, medical education in the United Kingdom is being refocused around general principles that could be expanded to other professions. The regulatory body, the General Medical Council, requires adherence to several concepts: preparation for lifelong learning, a shift from acquiring knowledge to acquiring clinical skills, an emphasis on communication and caring, and greater attention to ethical and legal issues. The Medical Schools Council is responding by updating curricula and teaching methods, professionalizing teaching, and carefully auditing the results.

In addition, the General Medical Council now explicitly requires that all medical undergraduates be made aware of a wide range of complementary and alternative therapies, how and why patients use them, and how they might affect patients' other treatments. All 33 British medical schools have informed Black that they are implementing this mandate in a variety of ways including through elective courses. At Bristol University, for example, medical students are taught the role of the fine arts in medicine, psychoneuroimmunology, and similar topics. Complementary and alternative medicine is presented as a model of care with a holistic approach. Students at Bristol may also elect to concentrate on the global environment in human health, where they consider climate change, water scarcity, mass migration, and food policy in health.

A survey of British graduate medical education indicates that these programs appear to be lagging in the incorporation of integrative medicine. The core curriculum for all 65 specialties includes requirements in such areas as communication, recognition of important risk factors, consideration of family history, and patient characteristics and preferences, and contains an attitude and behavior component that calls for the ability to show empathy for patients using complementary and alternative therapies, as well as for patients whose first language is not English. However, there is no explicit inclusion of integrative medicine or complementary and alternative medicine in the curricula. For example, the chair of the Joint Committee on Higher Surgical Training informed Black in January 2009 that "none of the surgical curricula contain any elements of complementary or alternative medicine."

Barriers to Change

Black noted that there are a number of barriers to reorienting the workforce to a more integrative approach to health. Competing demands for time and resources in health services and health professions training are formidable. Training the trainers can be difficult in the face of competing interests. Integrating the needs of patients with workforce competencies presents an enormous challenge that requires strong leadership.

Integrative health approaches also require a willingness to break free of professional silos. Overcoming these barriers is difficult, Black said, because the resistance to change and the immense authority of the status quo stand in the way; it is much easier to do nothing, especially in systems as complex as health care.

PANEL ON WORKFORCE AND EDUCATION

Panel Introduction
Elizabeth A. Goldblatt, Academic Consortium for
Complementary and Alternative Health Care

> *I am convinced that the progress or decline of humanity rests very largely with educators and teachers, who therefore have a tremendous responsibility. If you are a teacher, try not to merely transmit knowledge, but try at the same time to awaken your students' minds to basic human qualities such as kindness, compassion, forgiveness, and understanding.*
> *—Tenzin Gyatso, 14th Dalai Lama*

Goldblatt characterized education as the foundation of a compassionate and caring health care system and posed the question of what the role of education is in moving toward integrative medicine. The desire by people and patients for collaboration among their health care providers suggests a need to create innovative multidisciplinary educational experiences, training, and guidelines for all licensed health professionals.

In Goldblatt's view, this multidisciplinary approach is appropriate in the didactic, clinical, and research spheres—especially in clinical outcomes research, which can accommodate multifactorial approaches of integrative medicine. It also is relevant to the undergraduate, graduate, and continuing education levels, because training is needed at all levels to improve collaboration, teamwork, and the patient referral process.

The practice of truly integrative, patient-centered medicine requires interprofessional education, rather than educational silos, Goldblatt stated. Silos reinforce fragmentation and impede the collaboration that helps patients access combinations of treatments provided by diverse practitioners across disciplines. By contrast, collaborative education can serve to increase health professionals' knowledge of core competencies, which could include disease prevention, lifestyle change, diet, nutrition, exercise, stress reduction, environmental toxins, and issues in health policy—areas where most traditional education programs are weak, said Goldblatt. Collaboration also has been shown to increase patient satisfaction, improve health outcomes, and reduce costs.

As education changes, the workforce will change, Goldblatt said. The shortage of primary care practitioners could be alleviated, as the mantle of primary care is assumed not only by physicians but also by other competent practitioners, such as nurse practitioners, physician assistants, naturopaths, chiropractors, and traditional Chinese medicine practitioners, many of whom already serve as the first contact for patients in the health care system. The workforce also may change as the nation shifts to a focus on wellness rather than disease, and as providers regularly begin treatment with less invasive interventions before resorting to more invasive ones. Goldblatt echoed other participants in saying that our country needs to focus on health promotion and disease prevention. Education—at all levels—will have a key role in this fundamental shift.

Education Curricula
Mary Jo Kreitzer, University of Minnesota

Kreitzer expressed the view that shifting the focus of the health care system from disease to health requires new models of care—models that will use all appropriate licensed health care practitioners as primary care providers and allow them to practice to the highest and best use of their educations and capacities.

Educating heath professionals in integrative medicine is as daunting a task as transforming health care. The status quo is deeply entrenched as a result of the strength of traditional medicine in academia, said Kreitzer. Still, progress has been made in medical and nursing education, as integrative health content is being moved from elective to required core curricula. More graduate programs now offer specialization in integrative health; for example, the University of Minnesota is initiating a DNP degree (doctorate of nursing practice) in integrative health and healing. At the same time, educational institutions oriented to complementary and alternative medicine are expanding their course content on critical thinking and the role of evidence.

The National Center for Complementary and Alternative Medicine (NCCAM) has stimulated many of these changes. However, the necessary transformation in education requires shifts in content and process, and must go beyond the incremental changes that have been made so far, said Kreitzer. A shift in content could include an increased focus on health rather than the disease orientation that is currently used for educating biomedical professionals. The scope of training for both conventional providers and complementary and alternative practitioners is often narrow, failing to focus on health, wellness, nutrition, exercise, stress management, and other lifestyle issues, or on the social and environmental factors of health. Students are merely introduced to integrative therapies, without the necessary depth of exposure.

The process for education also needs to shift, Kreitzer reiterated. Education in silos hinders students' ability to quickly transition and adapt to a team environment. She pointed out that a range of providers is responsible for the care of the same patient in the same setting, yet there is almost no overlap in the education of those providers. Systematic interdisciplinary education is necessary for true collaboration.

According to Kreitzer, disruptive innovation is needed in both health professions education and health care delivery. Generally, innovation must come from outside, as leaders in a given field—whether in manufacturing, energy, or health care—tend to be victims and not initiators of disruption, due to their resistance to change and their failure to perceive its advances (Christensen et al., 2009). Faculty cultures in both traditional and nontraditional health professions are deeply ingrained and may be a barrier to change. Disruptive innovation must focus on the future vision of health care, emphasizing health instead of disease, a different mix of health professionals, a broader array of therapeutic approaches, and consumers who actively take charge of their health.

To match the health needs of the public, external investments in education should be predicated on innovation, Kreitzer said, and integrative health can provide the impetus for innovation. A new model of care suggests a different mix of health professionals, such as more nurse practitioners, physician assistants, and others to provide primary care, and a diminished focus on specialty care. A potential example of innovation could involve the 7,000 community health centers across the country that provide a medical home to indigent patients, furnish well-baby care, and fill other gaps in the health care system. Schools of nursing and complementary and alternative health professional training programs could partner with community health centers to create a comprehensive, holistic integrative model for health care. The American Recovery and Rein-vestment Act of 2009 included funding for the Health Resources and Services Administration (HRSA) to launch pilot projects that could be used to develop integrative health programs in the centers. In this way, "crisis would serve as a catalyst for reform," said Kreitzer.

Core Competencies
Victoria Maizes, University of Arizona

Maizes noted that *medical competence* is defined as the possession and use of the requisite knowledge, technical skills, and humanism (Jonsen, 1990). The word *competency* is derived from the Latin root *competere* and has three meanings. The first meaning is *to compete*, as in a race or game. The competent contestant was one who could run the race from start to finish. Maizes pointed out that educational leaders in integrative medicine have identified four domains of competence. First, integrative medicine practitioners should possess a broader set of knowledge, such as familiarity with nutritional recommendations for both specific conditions and optimal health, and knowledge about mind–body skills, physical activity, and spirituality. Second, practitioners should demonstrate a broader set of attitudes, such as awareness of how a practitioner's own personal, cultural, and spiritual beliefs affect his or her treatment recommendations, and an appreciation of the importance of self-care. Third, they should own a broader set of skills, such as the ability to communicate effectively with patients about all aspects of their health when taking a comprehensive health history. The fourth, and the final, domain reflects a second meaning of the Latin *competere* which is to *seek together*. It consists of a set of values that are timeless and relate to this deeper Latin meaning, and are exemplified by the dedication of the practitioner's own human experience to benefit patients.

Several model programs are now in place that incorporate these core competencies, noted Maizes. They exemplify another aspect of *seeking together*—namely, collaboration. One model is a 15-hour elective called The Healer's Art that was developed in the early 1990s by Dr. Rachel Naomi Remen at the University of California, San Francisco. This course is now taught to medical students in 70 medical schools, with plans to adapt it to nursing schools. The students write their own personal mission statement—in effect, their own personal Hippocratic Oath. An excerpt from a male medical student's oath reads:

> May you find in me the mother of the world. May
> my hands be a mother's hands, my heart be a
> mother's heart. May my response to your suffering
> be a mother's response to your suffering. May you
> know through our relationship that there is some-
> thing in this world that can be trusted.

Another model teaches clinicians to use the new patient-centered, decision-making tools that are emerging in health information technology. For example, Adjuvant! Online is a tool that assists breast cancer patients and their clinicians. Based on a woman's age, diagnosis, and pathology, the tool calculates the benefit of a specific hormonal therapy, such as tamoxofen, expressed in terms of a percentage reduction in the risk of a recurrence. When offered, for example, a 5 percent reduction, one woman may decide that this benefit is not worth the risks of the treatment, whereas another woman may feel the benefit is an opportunity to be seized. The tool facilitates patient–physician communication, patient-centered care, and informed decision making.

A third model is the Integrative Medicine in Residency (IMR) program developed at the Arizona Center for Integrative Medicine. IMR is being piloted, collaboratively, in eight residency programs around the country. IMR includes 200 hours of mandatory training and could eventually be applied to training programs for primary care physicians, specialty physicians, physician assistants, and nurse practitioner programs throughout the United States and abroad.

Maizes said that residency programs are the area within the medical education system that is most amenable to change, and they offer fertile ground for educating physicians in integrative medicine. Medical school curricula are packed, and it is in residency that physicians learn valuable practical skills. The number of trainees is typically small, offering an advantage to the use of a common online curriculum. Building evaluation into the system helps meet certification requirements. Maizes said that we have the opportunity to embody all the meanings of competency by finishing the task of building competency-based curriculum, seeking solutions together, and collaborating.

Interprofessional Education
Adam Perlman, University of Medicine and Dentistry of New Jersey

Perlman compared the progress of interprofessional education (IPE) to the stages of change model commonly referred to in behavior change interventions.[1] He noted that the time for advancing IPE from the contemplative and preparation stages to action has come. IPE is "any type of educational training, teaching, or learning session in which two or more health and social care professions are learning interactively" (Reeves et al., 2008). The need for IPE grows out of the fragmentation of modern health care, as patients are typically treated by multiple practitioners. Yet, these practitioners often do not communicate with each other adequately nor do they coordinate their services to assure quality care that is effective, efficient, and free of medical errors.

Perlman emphasized that the lack of IPE in physician education may render many physicians reluctant to collaborate or refer patients to other providers. For example, a primary care physician may resist discussing nutrition or acupuncture options with a patient, because these conversations may require time the physician does not have, information the physician is not familiar with or expert in, and possibly a referral to a provider with whom the physician is not acquainted.

To be most effective, Perlman said that IPE should be initiated early in the education and training process—in medical school, in the case of physicians. Students then can be introduced to other professions and begin to learn to work together effectively in teams. It is during the didactic phase of education that students in different disciplines can best develop shared values and master agreed-upon competencies. To facilitate this practical component of IPE, the curriculum must reflect the real-life experience of clinical teams, in order to prepare students for the dynamic environments they will be practicing in. Active learning methods must be implemented, including the use of simulated patients and clinical scenarios. Students should also learn how historical relationships among professions affect collaboration and where the frictions tend to occur.

Perlman described multiple challenges facing IPE, including the conventional medical mindset or culture, in which individual accomplishments are highly prized. Trained to find it and fix it, physicians are seldom rewarded for practicing effectively within teams. Lack of truly collaborative teams can reinforce professional territorialism, perhaps the

---

[1]Stages of change model includes five stages: precontemplation, contemplation, action, maintenance, and relapse (Prochaska and DiClemente, 1983).

greatest barrier to IPE. Differences in philosophy and language also create barriers between professions. Additionally, IPE is challenged by a lack of interdisciplinary, interinstitutional, and even interprogram relationships within schools.

In terms of research, IPE suffers from an overall dearth of well-developed studies and evidence. Most studies are small, most interventions are heterogeneous, and most methodologies are limited. Evidence is needed on the key elements of effective IPE, including skills and knowledge, but especially elements that influence attitudes. Models of best practice need to be developed in order to assess the effects of IPE on quality of care, service delivery, and patient satisfaction. Most importantly, Perlman said, an evidence base is needed for changing reimbursement policies to foster interprofessional collaboration in education, in research, and in the delivery of services to patients.

Workforce Reorientation
Richard A. Cooper, University of Pennsylvania

Cooper has developed projections of a large and critical nationwide shortage of physicians; a deficit of 200,000 physicians, approximately 20 percent of the needed supply, could arise by 2025. Because federal officials and other policy leaders maintain competing visions, current policies do not account for this shortage and provide no buffer against its likely effects, said Cooper. As a shortage comes to bear, the medical education pipeline, which can be up to 12 years in length, will prevent a quick response and remedy.

Signs of a shortage are already becoming apparent, Cooper said. Many physicians practicing in the United States are graduates of international medical schools, as U.S. medical schools fail to fill current needs. Many patients complain about long waits for appointments with a physician, or even about trouble finding a physician.

A rapidly escalating physician shortage would, like the recent collapse of the financial sector, produce a new reality unknown to any living American. Cooper said that it would upend many of the expectations expressed by previous speakers at the summit. Implicit in many of the speakers' prescriptions for change is the notion that physicians will play a crucial role in integrative medicine. However, in a shortage situation, physicians are likely to withdraw into "ever more narrow scientific and technological spheres, while other disciplines evolve to fill important gaps" (Cooper et al., 2002). In Cooper's view, physicians will continue to fill the specialty roles they are uniquely trained for, abandoning primary care and leaving it almost entirely to nonphysician providers. Cooper noted that the notion that future patients may experience regular 30-minute visits with a primary care physician is not credible in economic or personnel terms.

A long historical trend supports this prediction, he said. As physicians have fallen from almost one in three health care workers in the United States in 1920 to about 1 in 12 today, nurses and others have assumed tasks previously reserved to physicians. Until just a half-century ago, physicians resisted the notion that nurses could measure blood pressure. Yet today, nurses and other nonphysician health professionals do so routinely, and many are gaining broad competencies through doctorates and other graduate degrees. Their climb up the education ladder facilitates the shift away from physician dominance in performing health care functions. In short, Cooper said that physicians are sharing the platform of care with an expanding array of nonphysician clinicians, whose training and responsibilities are increasingly congruent with providing primary care.

Additionally, Cooper observed that specialty care is being redefined by technology and that primary care is an amalgam of wellness, prevention, and illness care. He suggested that a new workforce strategy be developed that includes economic and structural plans developed around the realities of the current situation. Society will have to determine the margins of personal and collective responsibility for primary care, as doing everything that primary care conceivably could do is not possible.

While there are many challenges to the current health care system, Cooper contended that the greatest challenge is poverty. People with the lowest 15 percent of income consume almost double the health care resources as people with the highest 15 percent of income. The health care crisis cannot be solved without coping with this major challenge.

Standards, Regulation, and Patient Safety
Cyril Chantler, The King's Fund

Chantler divided his remarks between two exhortations: *primum non nocere*, first do no harm, and *deinde adjuvare*, next do some good. To prevent harm, regulation of the practice of medicine was initiated in Europe and the United States in the 18th and 19th centuries. The regulatory scheme prohibited the unauthorized practice of medicine, which led to the criminalization of the practice of traditional or complementary medicine by nonphysicians. As recently as 1998, complementary medicine could be practiced in the Netherlands only by those who were medically qualified. In 2002, however, the World Health Organization recommended that governments adopt legislation and regulations for practice, education, training, and licensing in complementary medicine.

Chantler said that policy makers should assure that laws and regulations are truly necessary, and avoid overregulation that restricts innovation and increases costs; they should be proportionate, matching the degree of regulation to the extent that an activity can cause harm; and they should be enforceable. In the United Kingdom, physicians are regulated by the General Medical Council, which (like state boards of medical examiners in the United States) maintain a registry of physicians and can discipline physicians for ethical and other infractions. The General Medical Council also regulates osteopathic physicians, chiropractors, dentists, nurses, midwives, opticians, and pharmacists, while the Health Professions Council (HPC) covers 13 professions: art therapists, biomedical scientists, chiropodists/podiatrists, clinical scientists, dieticians, occupational therapists, operating department practitioners, orthoptists, paramedics, physiotherapists, prosthetists/orthotists, radiographers, and speech and language therapists. Legally, only those registered can use these titles.

The HPC is currently seeking to regulate herbalists, acupuncturists, Chinese medicinal practitioners, and clinical psychologists, but assimilating all modalities into the regulatory framework would be enormously expensive and cumbersome. As another means to distinguish a well-trained practitioner who subscribes to an ethical framework of practice, a new self-regulatory body, the Complementary and Natural Healthcare Council, has recently been established. All practitioners who wish to, and who provide evidence of their proper training and ethical and safe practice, may register with this new council.

Regulatory agencies are very competent at testing knowledge and responding to complaints, but, Chantler said, they are less adept at measuring clinical practice skills, such as surgical talent or ability in psychotherapy. He suggested that practitioners undertaking a specific technique, such as the Alexander technique in the management of chronic back pain, should all be held to the same standard of performance, regardless of profession.

Regulation has been viewed as necessary ever since Adam Smith famously observed, in *The Wealth of Nations*, that "[p]eople of the same trade seldom meet together, even for merriment and diversion, but the conversation ends in a conspiracy against the public." But, in *The Theory of Moral Sentiments*, Smith suggested that it is the conscience of the professional, not regulation, that provides the greatest protection to the public.

To do some good, Chantler said, the evidence base for complementary medicine should be built on effectiveness. While it is always desirable to understand the *efficacy* of an intervention—that is, whether an intervention works under ideal conditions, such as those of a clinical trial—it is possible to study the *effectiveness* of a treatment for patients in routine clinical care without having a full understanding of its efficacy. This may be particularly important with complex interventions that have psychological as well as pharmaceutical or physical components. Evaluation should ensure that a treatment is safe, beneficial, and cost-effective. The latter is especially important in establishing the value for public investment.

The evidence base, in Chantler's opinion, should include a combination of clinical outcomes, measures of patient satisfaction, and patient outcome measures, such as normal activities of daily living. It is imperative to know how well patients with chronic diseases are functioning over the course of time.

Most interventions, Chantler pointed out, now require integration—within and among different professions, different care modalities, and different locations, because much of the care provided takes place outside the hospital. This gives fundamental importance to maintaining an up-to-date and thorough medication record, including treatments provided through complementary modalities. Even if a single electronic health record for patients in all circumstances is not yet feasible, Web-based systems are being developed so that a contemporary summary can be made available to all practitioners involved in the patient's care. Chantler emphasized that integrative care requires such thorough communication.

Chantler concluded that, while the paramount concern is to ensure the patient's safety, the purpose of regulation is also to assure a high standard of care. Standards for professional competence should be clear and consistently applied, and outcomes, particularly patient outcomes, need to be measured, recorded, and audited. One important standard for the future will be the adequacy of teamwork and an assessment of how well health professionals communicate with each other.

Panel Discussion

Members of the panel responded to questions from the audience in a discussion moderated by Goldblatt. Selected points of discussion follow.

Collaborative Clinical Training

One question raised the issue of competence-based certifications for broadly defined practices, such as health-life coaching that could be undertaken by a variety of professions including health educators, nurses, and nutritionists. Maizes commented that people who train together often end up practicing together, so that interprofessional credentialing would be a logical extension of interprofessional education. Agreeing, Kreitzer suggested that community health centers can serve as both an integrated clinical site and a site for integrated education.

Incorporating Integrative Medicine into the Curriculum

Another question prompted further panel discussion on how to make integrative medicine part of the curriculum in medical schools, as well as in education programs for other health professions. Maizes suggested that it takes a champion within the school to promote the change. It also takes tools, such as a user-friendly program, with built-in evaluation, that meets applicable accreditation requirements. Kreitzer added that faculty development is needed, in order to help members of the entire faculty become comfortable with the presence of integrative medicine and be more accepting of a change in culture. The importance of faculty development has been demonstrated in the R25 educational grant program of the NCCAM.

Chantler noted that medical school deans are frequently asked to add new material to the curriculum. He also noted that the purpose of medical school is to provide education, with training to come afterward. He said that the education should include a common set of values, across professions, but the experience of interprofessional education is best placed at the graduate level. There, in residency programs, members of different professions can learn together, as they prepare to work together.

Physician Shortage

Asked to elaborate on issues of physician supply and distribution, Cooper stated that the physician shortage is mostly a matter of supply and demand—the population requiring health services is expanding, while new medical schools are not being built. A second major cause consists of advances in medicine and technology. Cooper noted that diseases that were once considered lethal, such as some forms of lung cancer, are now treatable, further increasing demand for physician services.

Regarding physician distribution, Cooper commented that the geographic distribution of physicians is not truly a maldistribution; physicians distribute themselves across the country in the same patterns as teachers and other professionals. Communities with more resources have more physicians and more teachers; that is a consequence of how our society distributes wealth, Cooper said.

Maizes challenged Cooper's formulation that primary care would not attract physicians in the coming years. As with end-of-life care, where skeptics who thought that hospice would be too expensive were proved wrong, primary care also can produce savings. Maizes said that the current model of care needs to evolve; it is based on outdated assumptions that most diseases are infectious diseases that require one-to-one clinical encounters. However, the chronic disease epidemic calls for a new model of care that emphasizes education and peer support that can be provided in a group visit with a team-based approach.

Achieving Interprofessional Education

Panel members were asked how to achieve interprofessional education in institutions that may not see the value of this type of education. Kreitzer stated that powerful countervailing incentives to encourage change in education are required in order to balance the skewed incentives of the current payment system. These forces could include accreditation agencies or federal grants for innovations. Maizes noted that graduate programs that offer training in integrative medicine often recruit more residents, and Perlman asserted that, ultimately, it comes down to leadership.

PRIORITY ASSESSMENT GROUP REPORT[2]

Dr. Aviad Haramati provided the report for the priority assessment group on reorienting the workforce. This summary includes the priorities discussed and presented by the assessment group to the plenary for its discussion and consideration; these priorities do not represent a consensus or recommendations from the summit.

Haramati began the report by putting education in context—all health professions' mission statements include some notion of training, knowledge, skill, compassion, and ethics. Yet, medical education generally misses the opportunity to reinforce the compassion of future physicians, the group suggested. One study indicated that empathy scores of University of Arkansas medical student cohorts declined steadily over the four years of medical education, as is shown in Figure 5-2 (Newton et al., 2008). Haramati remarked that students reflect the existing culture, and that the status quo is simply unacceptable.

The assessment group identified three top priorities: improving the workforce, academic curricula, and professional education. To improve the workforce, the assessment group suggested beginning with identifying the supply and distribution needs, as well as related data needs. This information will show whether the number of health professionals being trained reflects today's needs or for the demands that will develop over at least the next decade. Information gathering can start with building on what already has been done, as in geriatric team training.

To improve curricula, the designs of academic curricula should be examined to determine whether students are acquiring the necessary core competencies, skills, and attitudes required for meeting the future health needs of the population. Core competencies, including the ability to work in teams, need to be established through a national education dialog.

To improve professional education, the sphere of education should be widened to help current health professionals make the transition to integrative medicine, and to help patients assume more self-care. Primary

---

[2]See Chapter 1 for a description of the priority assessment groups. Participants on this assessment group included Victor Sierpina (moderator), Aviad Haramati (rapporteur), Adam Burke, Lee Chin, Timothy Culbert, Patrick Hanaway, Mary Jo Kreitzer, Roberta Lee, Karen Malone, Bill Meeker, and David Rakel.

care physicians and other integrative medicine practitioners should model behavior change for their patients, as well as build multiprofessional partnerships and educate patients in self-care. These activities can enrich primary care and make it more satisfying to physicians.

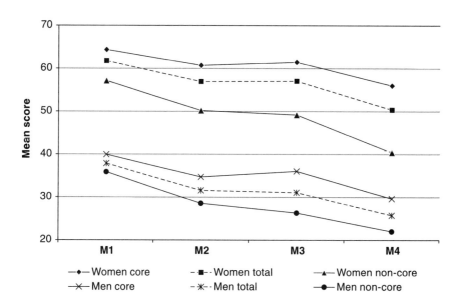

FIGURE 5-2 Decrease in empathy among medical students.

NOTES: Mean scores, by medical school year, specialty preference, and students' gender, for 419 men and women in the classes of 2001–2004, the University of Arkansas for Medical Sciences. Scores are for students' vicarious empathy (i.e., to have a visceral empathic response); responses were to a well-established measure of the various emotional qualities of empathy, administered at the beginning of each medical school year. The figure shows that vicarious empathy significantly decreased during medical education ($P < .001$), especially after the first and third years. Students choosing core careers had higher empathy than did those choosing noncore careers. Core refers to core specialties, (i.e., internal medicine, family medicine, obstetrics-gynecology, pediatrics, and psychiatry, which have greater patient contact), and *non*core refers to all other specialties, where patient contact is less.

SOURCE: Reprinted, with permission from *Academic Medicine*, Newton, B. W., L. Barber, J. Clardy, E. Cleveland, and P. O'Sullivan. Is there hardening of the heart during medical school? 83(3):244-249. Copyright 2008 Wolters Kluwer Health.

Key players are federal officials, especially in HRSA and the White House Office on Health Reform. Academic institutions, professional societies, and accrediting agencies also are involved, especially in curricular issues. Patient advocacy groups should help direct efforts in professional education.

Changes in education must happen quickly. The group identified 3-year goals that included development of economic incentives, which are essential to change the health care system; an interdisciplinary consensus on core competencies; and establishing national priorities for health care and health professions education. Academic institutions should recognize a responsibility to go beyond professional education and open their doors to educating the public.

The assessment group described a number of next steps that should be taken to advance the health service workforce. Convening key players, in all disciplines, in order to determine workforce needs is an important next step. Dialogue among stakeholder groups, including professional associations, educators, and academic institutions, must be increased. Finally, advocates of integrative medicine should make their voices heard, such as in academic journals.

6

Economics and Policy

*You can always count on Americans to do the
right thing once they have exhausted every other
possibility.*
—Winston Churchill

Senator Tom Harkin delivered the keynote address for the session on economics and policy. Harkin discussed the need for a more integrated approach to health care and what it will take to achieve it, and a panel moderated by Dr. Sean Tunis, represented the viewpoints of insurers, employers, and academia in discussing a range of financial and policy issues necessary for achievement of the visions of integrative medicine.

In leading off the summit discussion on economic and policy issues, Harkin noted the brightening prospects for comprehensive health reform. Echoing earlier observations, Harkin and Dr. Kenneth Thorpe reiterated that changes outside the health system (e.g., environmental and food policy) can have a profound effect on health, and reforms in these areas should also be considered and included in health reform discussions. Janet Kahn, among others, suggested greater coordination of health-promoting activities across government agencies, including agencies outside of the Department of Health and Human Services (HHS). Panelists cautioned that health reform, especially reform emphasizing integrative concepts, is far from a certainty. As a tactical matter, Tom Donohue warned against pointing fingers at other sectors and advised that advocates unite around commonly held values.

Dr. Reed Tuckson suggested that supporters of integrative approaches should not assume that health insurers will be opposed to their aims in the reform process. Similarly, unlike in previous attempts at health reform, Donohue said, businesses today are supportive of change. For insurers and the business community alike, the dominant concern is rising health care costs. Donohue and William George both viewed the business community as strong participants in reforming the health system, not only because of their traditional insurance role, but also because of their successes with employee wellness models. Some of the more successful models have not only improved employee health, but also have demonstrated return on investment to employers, as described by Dr. Kenneth Pelletier.

ECONOMICS KEYNOTE ADDRESS
Senator Tom Harkin, U.S. Senate (D-IA)

Integrative health care is finally coming to prominence in the United States. For a number of reasons that Harkin noted, the timing for reform seems to be right. Harkin recalled that a few days prior to the summit, President Obama, before a joint session of Congress, predicted that Congress would pass a comprehensive health reform measure this year and that the centerpiece of that reform would be a new emphasis on prevention and wellness.

Harkin observed that Washington has been transformed by new energy and a new sense of purpose, and in no area of public policy is this more dramatic than in health reform.[1] Congress is also moving forward energetically; Sen. Edward Kennedy, chair of the Senate Health Committee, has established a set of working groups to help shape the Senate's health reform bill. Harkin heads the working group on prevention and public health, which focuses on wellness, disease prevention, and strengthening the public health infrastructure. On the day prior to his presentation, Harkin chaired a hearing on how health reform legislation could be the vehicle to move the nation forward in integrative medicine and to create a culture of wellness. All these signals together, he said, create momentum not just to pass health reform, but to pass "the right kind of health reform."

Currently, payment incentives are biased toward providing conventional medical care—patching and fixing people when they get sick, said Harkin. In medicine, what is reimbursed the most is practiced the most; and what is practiced the most is taught in medical schools, thus perpetuating the cycle. Meanwhile, alternative therapies, preventive strategies, and integrative health approaches are often marginalized.

It is time to think anew, he said, time to "disenthrall ourselves from the dogmas and the biases that have made our current health system in so

---

[1] Harkin noted that he preferred the term *health reform*, rather than *health care reform*, because he believes the changes needed are fundamental and systemwide, not merely related to reimbursement.

many ways wasteful and dysfunctional." Harkin said that this requires a system that emphasizes care coordination and continuity, patient-centeredness, holistic approaches, and wellness. Such an integrative approach takes advantage of the very best scientifically based practices, whether conventional or alternative. It focuses on improving health outcomes and has great potential to reduce health care costs.

Harkin's belief in the potential value of integrative approaches dates back many years. In 1992, he authored legislation that created the Office of Alternative Medicine at the National Institutes of Health. In 1998, he sponsored legislation to elevate the office to what is today the National Center for Complementary and Alternative Medicine, which one summit participant suggested could be renamed the National Institute for Integrative Health Care. Harkin said that the country now faces an historic opportunity, and "We've got to get it right." He cited Dr. Mark Hyman's statement in a recent hearing that "we need to rethink not just the way we do medicine, but also the medicine we choose to do."

Another factor that makes such an ambitious effort timely is that today, unlike previous attempts at reform, there is broad agreement among ordinary Americans, corporate America, and health care providers that the status quo is disfunctional, wasteful, and increasingly intolerable, said Harkin. The scope of health reform that Harkin envisions would go beyond merely providing health insurance coverage or finding new health services payment methods, important as those issues are. He noted that *what* we are paying for is as important as *how* we are paying for it: "It makes no sense just to figure out a better way to pay the bills for a system that is broken and unsustainable." He said that a reformed system should implement a national prevention and wellness structure; offer a pragmatic, integrative approach to health care; and base reimbursement on outcomes and quality rather than quantity. Without this orientation, any reform effort will fail the American people, he said.

Health reform should touch many aspects of people's lives, especially outside the health sector. Harkin noted that health reform must encompass health and include consideration for providing better nutrition in schools and exercise opportunities in the built environment, such as sidewalks and bike paths; it should encourage wellness programs in workplaces and community centers; it should provide opportunities for wellness services, exercise, stress reduction, and socialization in our senior centers; and it should make widely available the informational, screening, and counseling programs that help people take charge of their own health. Harkin also chairs the Senate Agriculture Committee, which this year will consider reauthorization of the Child Nutrition Bill. It, too, can contribute to health reform by ensuring that school children have healthier food choices.

If, as Andrew Weil says, the default status of the body is to be healthy, then the default status of public policy should be to facilitate that natural process and promote health and prevention, commented Harkin. Physicians and a full range of other health care professionals, as well as teachers, physical trainers, counselors, and others, all have a role to play in assuring both the physical and mental health of our population. Good mental health is critical to good physical health and well-being, said Harkin; any number of physical ailments start, often in childhood, with mental, emotional, or behavioral problems—stress, lack of emotional support, addiction. These problems may worsen over time and, left untreated, have serious consequences for health, relationships, educational attainment, life skills, and work performance.

Harkin reaffirmed his commitment to do all he can to change the nation's health system and place integrative health care at the heart of the 2009 health reform efforts. He encouraged summit participants to follow the debates and discuss these issues with family, friends, and colleagues. He added a note of caution:

> Just because integrative health care is the most commonsense, rational, health-effective, and cost-effective approach to reform, does not mean it is a done deal. Nothing in this town is done easily, and there are tremendous entrenched forces and vested interests that will defend the conventional allopathic medicine with all their power.

The kind of reform he envisions will not happen unless people speak up for it; he emphasized that everyone is a key player in supporting these efforts, so his message is "Seize the day."

Discussion

Following the keynote presentation, several members of the audience offered their thoughts on how the current health reform discussion could be shaped to advance integrative medicine and improve the health of the nation.

Nutrition and Children's Health

The first participant, a nutritionist, asked about the possibility of including in the child nutrition bill a requirement that schools have hygienic, operable water fountains, so that water could be a healthy alternative to sugar-laden soft drinks. Another participant suggested increased emphasis on reducing high-fructose corn syrup and increasing omega-3 fatty acids in the American diet.

Harkin, who has worked to get healthier foods into schools and eliminating unhealthy choices from school vending machines, recognized the participants concern and described one pilot program that was introduced in the 2001 Farm Bill. The program was designed to ensure that children had freely available fresh fruits and vegetables throughout the school day, not just at lunch. The program began with a $4 million budget and was implemented in 100 schools across four states. It has been wildly successful with school administrators, parents, and students, and with Harkin's leadership the program was expanded to $1 billion in the most recent Farm Bill. Over the next five years 90 percent of students enrolled in free or reduced lunch programs will have access to free fresh fruits and vegetables.

Comparative Effectiveness

The recent economic stimulus legislation included funds to support comparative effectiveness research for health care practices, and several participants iterated the importance of including integrative approaches in these comparisons. Harkin emphasized that the goal of this research is to reduce the cost of the health care system and improve quality and outcomes of care. He noted that the research will not just look at the current system and approaches to care, but that it will also look at other modalities that are available, such as those described by Ornish. Ideally, the results of this type of research will provide information and evidence that can be used by individuals in the decisions they make about their own care.

PANEL ON ECONOMICS AND POLICY

Panel Introduction
Sean Tunis, Center for Medical Technology Policy

Panel moderator Tunis noted that his background is not in integrative medicine but that his past work as chief medical officer for Medicare and current work as head of the Center for Medical Technology Policy has made him a realist. He reiterated Harkin's statement that just because health reform and its inclusion of integrative approaches make sense, does not mean it is inevitable—such significant changes will face formidable challenges.

Tunis said that summit participants should take the opportunity to become effective advocates, to engage in the debate, and to focus their energies on the most promising avenues for change. Many aspects of potential health reforms will affect the future of integrative health care. For example, reforms that tie reimbursement to outcomes will reflect not just how much practitioners do, but the extent to which their contribution actually improves patient outcomes. When financial incentives are set, someone, at some point, will define which patient outcomes matter. Tunis said that integrative health care practitioners will want to be part of that critical discussion. Generally, Tunis observed, integrative medicine has been absent during the push toward comparative effectiveness research, and advocates for integrative health care need to work to assure that integrative approaches receive adequate attention as this type of research moves forward.

Tunis noted that this panel was designed to explore the challenges and the solutions, mechanisms, strategies, and tactics that will help ensure that integrative health care becomes a key component of a newly reformed health system.

Economic Burden of Chronic Disease
Kenneth Thorpe, Emory University

Thorpe opened with an array of statistics that exemplify challenges in the current health reform debate. He noted that three-fourths of U.S. health care spending is for patients with one or more chronic conditions, which makes these disorders a prime target in efforts to improve the quality and affordability of care. Obesity rates in the United States have doubled since the mid-1980s; this increase alone accounts for about 30 percent of the subsequent growth in health care spending and costs about $220 billion a year. Further, for every dollar we spend on medical care costs linked to chronic illnesses, we lose another $4 in productivity. While heart disease caused the largest increase in Medicare costs between 1987 and 1997, it is no longer even in the top five cost contributors, which are: diabetes, asthma, pulmonary conditions, arthritis, and back problems—health problems, like heart disease, that can, in many cases, be linked to personal lifestyle.

Thorpe observed that, with this president and this session of Congress, there is a greater opportunity to put together a coordinated, *administration-wide* policy on prevention. Currently, numerous unconnected and uncoordinated programs operated by HHS and other federal agencies offer different ways to intervene to promote health and prevent disease. Organizing these programs in a coherent, thoughtful way could have a tremendous cumulative impact.

To improve health care outcomes and reduce costs for the large number of Americans with chronic conditions requires actions outside the traditional physician's office. Thorpe noted that today's patient populations and their clinical characteristics are very different than when Medicare was enacted, and many of the services patients need most are not necessarily services that must be provided by a physician. However, the reimbursement system is based on benefits designed four or five decades ago and does not accommodate these needs. Policy makers must figure out how to encourage and cover both nonphysician services and team-based care, said Thorpe.

Large systems, like the Mayo Clinic, Geisinger, and Kaiser Permanente have solved some of these problems. However, most Americans do not obtain their health care through sophisticated, integrated group practices. In fact, more than 80 percent of U.S. physicians practice in ones and twos, and these small practices account for about 40 percent of the nation's primary care capacity. Thorpe said that strategies must be devised to transfer to the small-office setting some of the functionality and useful components that make those large models effective. Senator Baucus, for example, is focusing on delivery system innovations. One model under consideration is to assemble community health teams that include nurse practitioners, social workers, behavioral health workers, and nutritionists that can collaborate with an area's small physician practices and provide care coordination, primary prevention, and community-based outreach services. Lessons can also be learned from innovative state-level approaches to reform such as those in Vermont, North Carolina, Rhode Island, and Pennsylvania. These models frequently factor in community-based prevention strategies and small physician practices.

Insurer Perspective
Reed V. Tuckson, UnitedHealth Group

Tuckson reminded summit participants that health insurance companies such as UnitedHealth Group have agendas and missions that are well aligned with the summit's goals. Many insurance companies work hard to ensure responsible policies for prevention, wellness, and integrated care, he said. In fact, UnitedHealth Group views itself as "a health and well-being company"; for example, the company spends millions of dollars to collect and analyze data, in order to identify individuals' risk factors for disease, then provide them with a variety of individually tailored support services to assist in personally appropriate preventive interventions. It also uses its data to identify gaps in care; conducts sophisticated analyses to assure that individuals have received appropriate care; provides evidence-based guidance to individuals through their preferred electronic or print vehicles; and facilitates access to health coaching from trained clinicians. Tuckson said that these are just some elements of the company's patient-centered care capabilities that are devoted to enhancing health and wellness for each individual.

From an insurer's perspective, one of the most significant barriers to expanding integrated health care is the unsustainable escalation in health care costs. One major contributor to that cost escalation, he said, is "Everyone wants everything all the time." As more people experience preventable chronic illnesses, as increasingly expensive pharmaceuticals and technologies are developed, and as consumer demand remains insatiable, health care costs will continue to be challenging, according to Tuckson. Financing for new interventions and for services associated with integrative medicine will present new challenges, he said, especially until researchers produce convincing evidence of clinical and cost-effectiveness. Concerns about the quality of current clinical care delivery form an equally challenging context for the introduction of integrative medicine, said Tuckson. Research indicates that almost half of clinical care delivery today is inconsistent with prevailing evidence-based guidelines. In the case of new (often expensive) technologies, the criteria for clinical appropriateness are often weak, and deviation from the available evidence is a frequent concern, noted Tuckson. Additionally, at an alarming rate, individuals fail to exercise personally appropriate health protecting and enhancing behavior; almost 21 percent of the population continues to smoke; the incidence of diabetes is increasing rapidly; and the prevalence of obese children is such that 32 percent of children and teens are overweight and 16 percent are obese.

Within this context, in order to gain acceptance for integrative health care, advocates must have a realistic organizing vision for what they are trying to achieve, how integrative services will be implemented, what the roles and scopes of practice are of key disciplines, and what the evaluation criteria are, said Tuckson. Decisions regarding the incorporation of proposed interventions must inevitably be grounded in evidence of effectiveness, and arguments about the difficulty of accumulating this evidence will not lessen the importance of this critical information. Advancing integrative health care will also require answers to a series of critical questions that Tuckson posed to the plenary session:

- Who pays for prevention? What are the relative roles of public, private, and individual resources?
- How can population-based prevention efforts be effectively coordinated with individual preventive initiatives? How can synergies be maximized?
- Should the staffing of new patient-centered multidisciplinary preventive care be static or fluid to meet case-by-case challenges?
- How are different members of the comprehensive care team trained, credentialed, evaluated, coordinated and reimbursed? What are ways to prevent redundancy and maximize efficiency?
- What is the health return for employers' investments in integrative health care?

Finally, Tuckson said that the new integrative health team will require new coding systems in order to capture the services they deliver and new health information technology infrastructures that can record and enable assessment of their work on behalf of the unique needs of individuals.

Tuckson concluded his remarks by committing UnitedHealth Group to actively participate in the exploration of the questions noted above, particularly those related to acquiring the evidence necessary for advancing this important field.

Business Community Perspective
Thomas J. Donohue, U.S. Chamber of Commerce

The U.S. Chamber of Commerce represents three million companies, which gives the organization a strong interest in health care. The main health care concern for the business community today is that health care simply costs too much, especially for the growing number of retirees, said Donohue. Thorpe said that Medicare patients are different today than in the mid-1960s, and there are a lot more of them, said Donohue. When Medicare was enacted, actuaries estimated the average American's lifespan at 62.5 years. Now, Americans who reach 65 live nearly two more decades, on average. This puts a tremendous strain on companies with growing numbers of retirees, and it creates serious dislocations in industries that employ far fewer people than they used to in order to accomplish the same—and more—work.

The fundamental change needed in this country, particularly for health care, is to stop blaming everyone else, said Donohue. The problems of our current system are not caused by health care providers or the insurance companies. "We are only willing to pay them so much, and as Reed indicated, we want every service available to man," he said. To successfully move forward, everyone—corporations, hospitals, doctors, professional practitioners of every type, and insurance companies—must be involved in the reform debate.

The best strategy, he said, may be to identify and unite around common issues that everyone agrees to and can support. Wellness is one. Another is the need for serious health information technology, not only to find out which treatments work, what the best practices are, and where people get the best results, but also to run complex health care systems. Most important, he said, almost everyone can agree that there has to be a way to cover people who do not have health insurance, because care for uninsured people is being provided at an unnecessarily high cost.

Yet, there are issues where agreement will not come easily, including how to divide finite health care dollars. Donohue said that every advocacy group should understand that "You are a petitioner. You want your piece of the pie. The biggest thing we all have to worry about . . . is, how much pie is there? How much pie can we afford?" He cautioned that society cannot bear the cost of a grossly expensive system created by petitioners, and that infighting cannot be allowed to negatively affect the issues having widespread support.

Donohue predicted that the business community will ultimately be supportive during the upcoming reform debates, because businesses are under severe pressure to change the status quo. In fact, he said, business can be a strong partner in reform efforts, building on the strengths of the employer-based health insurance system, which covers some 150 million Americans. Another strength offered by business is the investment many employers have made to develop a healthier workforce. They understand that healthier workers are more productive and reduce the employer's short- and long-term medical costs. Donohue noted that the nation's diverse workplaces are useful laboratories for experimentation with new models of care and are contained environments for measuring results.

Because of the employer-based system's record of innovation, measurement capacity, and motivation to achieve many of the wellness objectives described at the summit, Donohue supports continuation of the employer-based insurance system over a single-payer model.

Employer Perspective
William W. George, Harvard Business School

George said "The employer-based system is the strongest part of our health care system," and that integrative health care is the key to its future. In fact, George said that it will not be possible to offer health insurance to 100 percent of Americans unless we have a health system that promotes wellness and prevention.

George noted his belief that employers have a role and responsibility in health promotion and disease prevention. Employers—especially those in the health care field, which in many communities are the area's largest employers—should serve as role models for customers and patients. Ways to do this include hospital food services that offer only healthy choices and no-smoking policies that cover a health facility's entire property, including parking lots. The goal for employers that emphasize wellness is not achieving the lowest cost; it is to have 100 percent of employees fully present on the job every day—in other words, improved productivity.

Company CEOs need to take initiative and active leadership on health care matters and not delegate them to unions, health plans, or company benefits managers, said George. Instead, business leaders need to invest time on health care issues, make serious attempts to reduce paperwork that drives up costs, and recognize that employee health is tightly linked to company strategy and productivity goals. As an example, he said that Target stores find a direct correlation between the health of their employees and customer satisfaction. The stores where employees are healthiest have the highest customer satisfaction ratios, as well as the greatest revenue growth.

George also said that business leaders need to devise ways to engage employees in their health and empower them to take responsibility for it. The full range of wellness services that employees need starts with a corporate culture where health is something that is honored and enjoyed. This culture could include having nutritionists on staff whom employees can talk to as necessary; offering stress management options, support groups, and health coaches; and having a fitness center. These are not "perks," he said—they are services that are important to health, and the workplace is one of the most convenient places to offer them. He also suggested that a great deal of support can be provided online with social networking, and that this support should be made fun.

Employees who are pregnant or have chronic conditions may require additional support and active management, some of which can be provided at work, said George. When employees need hospitalization, the employer should encourage treatment in designated centers of excellence, because of the direct correlation between volume and quality of care and, therefore, long-term costs.

Even with all these employer-provided options, the basic premise still must be that employees are responsible for their health. George said that the role of employers is to give employees the resources and, perhaps, even provide financial incentives for wellness. For example, employers could offer incentives for maintaining a healthy weight, healthy cholesterol levels, or practicing healthy behavior, like not smoking.

If employers took on these suggested roles, there would not need to be as many government health reforms, said George, although government should require portability of health plans, so that when people change jobs they can take their health plan with them if they choose. George supported pretax health insurance coverage for every American and development of private insurance pools for small groups of employees, employees without health coverage, and the unemployed, so that everyone can have access to health opportunities typically offered by large companies.

In conclusion, George also warned against blaming others, described by Donohue. Rather, he endorsed making integrated health care the core of our nation's system and building on employer capacity, "so that wellness and prevention become the essential characteristic of every workplace in America."

Behavior Change Incentives and Approaches
Janet R. Kahn, Integrated Healthcare Policy Consortium

Kahn began by building on prior discussions of summit speakers and participants, noting that a broad range of disciplines is involved in integrative care. For true integration, these diverse practitioners must be knowledgeable about and respectful of one another's expertise and collaborate effectively in the interest of their patients, said Kahn. Integrative health care need not depend solely on doctors to do patient-oriented, mind–body care; rather, it should take full advantage of the existing experiential base of qualified providers.[2] This would allow patients real choice about the kind of provider they use. Moreover, making better use of the full range of providers who can serve in a primary care role— nurse practitioners, physician assistants, naturopathic physicians, and others—would help reduce the current primary care physician shortage.

In Vermont, for example, naturopathic physicians are now classified as primary care providers and are reimbursed by Medicaid, providing the opportunity for a natural experiment. In general, states' authority to set scope-of-practice laws produces interstate differences in practice patterns, providing a valuable opportunity for comparative research on mechanisms for delivering primary care services.

At the federal level, Kahn said that a single entity should be responsible for coordinating integrative health-related policy efforts across agencies, perhaps through an Office of Integrative Health Care and Wellness. That office could be charged with scoring domestic policy proposals—not just those within HHS, but across the executive branch, including those related to education, transportation, the environment, housing, and agriculture—as to their potential impact on health and illness, just as the Congressional Budget Office scores the potential financial impact of all proposed legislation.

---

[2]Kahn noted that the term *qualified* refers to providers who are licensed and have been educated at institutions that are accredited by a Department of Education-recognized accrediting body.

Kahn noted that social scientists have demonstrated that it is relatively easy to enhance someone's knowledge about a behavioral health risk and slightly more challenging to help them shift their attitudes toward it, but that getting someone actually to change their behavior can be very difficult. Individuals have to decide not to smoke or not to eat junk food, not once or twice, but multiple times daily. There is no one best way to accomplish successful behavior change for everyone. Even with solid evidence of effectiveness for such interventions as smoking cessation, potential program sponsors need to know exactly how such programs should be implemented for their target population, and what their return on investment will be, said Kahn.

Clearly, health professionals do not change other people's behavior—individuals must change their own behavior. However, health professionals can promote these changes with policies, incentives, and media messages that persuade people they *want* to change. While individuals do the hard work of changing what they eat and how they exercise, health professionals can provide emotional support for the individual trying to change, whether they achieve their goals or not. If they did not do it this time, they might the next.

Opportunities to facilitate behavior change are all around us. People are social beings embedded in networks—from preschools to workplaces to retirement homes—and health professionals should work in those networks to encourage behavior change. Also, people live in both natural and built environments that are dramatically different across the country and vary across class lines. These environments can be improved to make exercise easier or healthier food more available.

The workplace offers many possibilities for behavior change, including a wide range of incentives and rewards, such as those previously described. Incentives in the workplace do work and can offer an opportunity for cost containment. Kahn noted that some companies have been able to reduce their annual increase in health care costs to 1 percent, rather than the average 8 or 9 percent. But incentives can backfire, Kahn warned. Some employees may feel that these incentives, which require the regular collection of health information, impinge on their privacy. Workplaces that have been most successful have coupled financial incentives with team building and social support for behavioral change.

Central to success of behavior change strategies, whether across society or within a single workplace, is the use of multiple message channels and the alignment of these messages with policies. Kahn cited smoking cessation as an imperfect, but highly successful effort at health behavior change. In the United States in 1965, roughly 51 percent of men and 34 percent of women smoked. By 2005, rates of smoking dropped to 24 percent of men and 18 percent of women. Interventions that facilitated this change involved a coordinated health policy effort that included approaches ranging from increased taxes on cigarettes, to municipal regulation of where people could and could not smoke, to nicotine patches and workplace smoking cessation programs.[3]

Within a corporation or within a country, policy makers should not be talking about health and wellness on one hand while creating situations that lead to unhealthy behavior on the other, said Kahn. On the provider side, financial incentives encourage use of expensive interventions rather than prevention strategies. Incentives encourage medical students to pursue specialty rather than primary care careers. Equally powerful incentives for prevention and health should be purposefully reset, she said.

The goal, suggested Kahn, is to encourage people to want to change their behavior, and then to be prepared to help them when the point of wanting to change. This requires a state of readiness on the part of the employer, public health system, health care providers, and others, and this involves both removing barriers to change and having programs and systems that can provide necessary support. One aspect of this can be incentives that can make change worth it in multiple ways including financially and socially. To make healthy behavior normative, Kahn said, incentive structures must be aligned, not working at cross-purposes.

Rewards of Integrative Medicine
Kenneth R. Pelletier, University of Arizona School of Medicine and University of California (UCSF) School of Medicine

Analyzing the economics of integrative medicine defies easy economic analysis. When people approach such a difficult topic, they tend to turn to tools like cost–benefit analysis, with its aura of precision, said Pelletier. Cost–benefit analysis is a complex field with perhaps a dozen different alternative methods, all of which can provide useful information. These include cost–benefit analysis, cost-effectiveness analysis,

---

[3]Kahn noted that Dr. Kenneth Warner, Dean of the School of Public Health at the University of Michigan, has authored a chapter entitled "Tobacco Policy in the U.S.: Lessons for the Obesity Epidemic" describing coordinated approaches to improving health (Mechanic et al., 2005).

assessment of net present value, return on investment, and econometric modeling, which can encompass all of the previous techniques.

Different cost–benefit methodologies reflect different perspectives. They often result in incomparable and even nongeneralizable outcomes. A systematic review conducted by Pelletier and colleagues provided several insights about these differences as they apply to integrative medicine (Pelletier et al., unpublished). Researchers examined all the definitions of the patient-centered medical home, chronic care management, extended primary care, and integrative medicine, and found that the various definitions have more in common than not. One of the distinguishing factors of integrative medicine was that, in the majority of definitions, it included evidence-based alternative medicine.

The researchers decided to examine what cost–benefit analysis would look like when applied to this distinguishing characteristic. They conducted an international literature search that yielded 59 cost–benefit analyses, 39 of which were considered full evaluations. From these, they identified eight alternative medicine modalities that appeared to be cost-effective in treating various conditions, including acupuncture, guided imagery, relaxation, and various forms of meditation. One specific cost-effective modality/condition pair was use of acupuncture for migraine. While integrative medicine is clearly not synonymous with complementary and alternative medicine (CAM), this research showed that there are CAM components that are likely to be cost-effective in an integrative care model.

Pelletier has dedicated time to managing clinical trials in various worksites, and he noted that corporations are perfect sites for implementing and evaluating integrative medicine. First, employers call people *people* not *patients*. He said that corporations have a vested interest in the health, performance, and well-being of their employees, while they have no vested interest in disease. Additionally, employers are not wedded to certain modalities of treatment, as long as it is effective in terms of clinical and cost outcomes. If, for example, an employer learns that acupuncture for back pain is superior to surgery, they would support the use of acupuncture.

Pelletier reported on research that identified 153 clinical and cost outcome studies of worksite integrative health approaches (Pelletier, in press), all of which have demonstrated net benefits in terms of short-term and long-term disability, absenteeism, general retention, key personnel retention, productivity, performance, and presenteeism.[4] Of the 63 studies that used cost–benefit analyses, all but one older study showed positive results, and 24 reported a return on investment—the hard-to-reach measure that is the gold standard within the business community.

The most conservative return-on-investment result that would be considered positive is 1:1. Many people in a corporate environment would be very happy with a dollar-spent:dollar-value-recouped return, he said. But the returns on investment found in this literature ranged from 3.5–4.9:1. These are salient results, because the return on investment does not have to be very high for the dollar savings to be large. Pelletier also noted that, on average, rate of return outcomes were most evident after approximately 3.25 years, suggesting that these types of employer investments should be long term.

The potential for such persuasive results indicates that cost–benefit analyses should be included in assessments of integrative medicine programs, especially effectiveness trials. Pelletier predicted that integrative medicine and its preventive components will prove to be dramatically more cost-effective than many conventional services, at least on a purely empirical basis. He also agreed with Donohue and George that employers have a large stake in both ensuring employee health and involvement in health and medical care reform.

Pelletier said that within 2 to 3 years it should be possible to create a minimum set of standardized measures that could be used to assess any and all health services that purport to be safe, effective, and cost-beneficial. This would provide a basis for more accurate comparison of integrative and conventional care approaches. The problem in the nation's medical care sector, which currently spends $2.5 trillion annually, is not that it needs more money. The problem is that these resources are misallocated, he said, because many of the services and interventions that are regularly paid for would not pass any of the measures of cost-effectiveness. By conducting appropriate cost–benefit analyses, Pelletier said it will be possible to create an evidence base for allocating health care resources in a more scientific and cost-effective way.

---

[4]*Presenteeism* measures the ability of a person to be present at work, both physically and mentally.

Panel Discussion

Members of the panel responded to questions from the audience in a discussion moderated by Tunis, who began the discussion by repeating what he called "a great truism about Washington," which is that when everyone seems to agree on any policy idea, it usually means it has not been defined specifically enough. Tunis noted that the summit had engendered much agreement on what needs to be done to promote the adoption of integrative health care, and he encouraged participants to dive into some of the details.

Evidence for Integrative Medicine

Participants asked how much and what kinds of additional evidence would be needed to make integrative health care approaches more widely accepted. Given how much evidence had been presented at the summit, it seemed to some participants that there should be more forward progress in terms of adopting and reimbursing clearly effective programs.

One of the accomplishments of the summit is that it made available some of these studies, Tuckson said. Much of the research presented is not well known outside the integrative medicine community. He said that it needs to be examined closely and then disseminated more widely. Because so few people are familiar with this body of research, they will challenge it, Tuckson warned, and it must meet the scientific scrutiny that should be applied to all interventions.

Obtaining definitive evidence about prevention can be difficult and can require a significant amount of time. However, when it comes to prevention and wellness, George said, we simply cannot wait for randomized trials to prove that modalities such as meditation and fitness and diet and nutrition work. He noted that there is evidence to support them now, and they should be put into practice and measured after the fact. "This may not fit the pure scientific model," he said, but if you can show employers cost–benefit data after the fact, they will continue supporting these programs.

Evidence for Conventional Care

Another participant countered that much of conventional, allopathic medicine has never been proved effective, yet billions of dollars are spent on it, creating an evidentiary double-standard.

According to Tuckson, the most important driving force in the health care industry today is performance assessment. Anyone associated with organizing or paying for health care benefits is frustrated with the variability in quality of care, he said. This is especially important to patients, as they increasingly are expected to participate actively in selecting the physicians and hospitals they use. This scrutiny creates enormous tension in the allopathic community, Tuckson said, but ultimately, these efforts will lead to a much closer connection between reimbursement and performance. Moving forward, the system will need to find performance measures that emphasize outcomes more than process. Although this field is not very mature yet, it is moving rapidly.

Integrative Medicine and Models of Reimbursement

A participant described the difficulty in obtaining full reimbursement for the integrative medicine services she provides. Tunis said that her question raises the issue of whether a reformed system would approach integrative services in the old fee-for-service way or adopt some alternative.

Worksites have developed some generalizable alternative models, Pelletier said, that work in the community and draw on community resources. These models are entirely dependent on networks of providers. For example, Cisco Systems recently built a patient-centered medical home within its corporate headquarters that is linked to day care and corporate health services. It includes evidence-based alternative medicine, uses an electric medical record, and has an on-site pharmacy. Use of the Internet for telemedicine applications also will enable some interesting hybrid approaches, as will use of health coaches to reach out into the community.

When it comes to reimbursement, Pelletier said he would advocate very strongly for adequate compensation for primary care. Reimbursement problems continue to be difficult, Tuckson acknowledged, saying, "Let's be excited about trying to answer [the questioner] in a way that is affordable and sustainable to the health system and fair to practitioners."

PRIORITY ASSESSMENT GROUP REPORT[5]

Helen Darling provided the report of the priority assessment group that focused on the economic incentives of integrative medicine. This summary includes the priorities discussed and presented by the assessment group to the plenary session for its discussion and consideration; these priorities do not represent a consensus or recommendations from the summit.

In discussing this area, the group decided that its first priority relates to the big picture: figuring out how to go from an unhealthy to a healthy America. This means not only determining the steps that need to be taken, but also deciding which ones society wants to pay for collectively. The summit discussions have described many valuable types of treatment, supported by a growing body of evidence, yet many are not covered benefits under most insurance plans so are not reimbursed fully (if at all), and must be paid for by the consumer.

The second priority identified by the group was the need for an orderly, ongoing process to make decisions related to which new integrative services will be reimbursed. It is not enough to assert that insurance should pay for these services, since the public, through premiums, taxes, or lower wages, is the ultimate payer. We have to somehow decide together what services are safe, effective, cost-effective, and have added value. Care delivery needs to be organized better, possibly through team-based approaches, and paid for based on outcomes, not just individual services. The group suggested that perhaps teams can be paid on a capitated basis, enabling them to decide how to produce the most health for society's investment. To bring appropriately trained people into teams may require programs like one in Washington State that provides loan forgiveness for integrative care practitioners who serve 3 years in underserved communities, as one participant in the group suggested.

The third priority was to consider integrative medicine a solution, not an add-on. Reimbursement decisions are difficult, and not every service, intervention, or modality of care can be paid for. If the system does not identify low-value, wasteful, or harmful services to eliminate, it cannot recoup the nearly $400 billion needed to provide coverage for the currently uninsured population. However, the push for cost-control may turn

---

[5]See Chapter 1 for a description of the priority assessment groups. Participants on this assessment group included Sean Tunis (moderator), Helen Darling (rapporteur), Eric Caplan, Robert DeNoble, Erminia Guarneri, Patricia Herman, Davis Masten, Anne Nedrow, William Rollow, Richard Sarnat, and Michelle Simon.

out to be a strong incentive to adopt integrative approaches, particularly if Americans understood that these approaches are being advocated not because they cost less, but because they produce superior results.

The group's fourth priority was to incentivize organizations outside the health care sector—schools, communities, employers, and consumers—to provide effective care, defined broadly. This is a way to reallocate existing resources to achieve greater health benefit.

Key roles in achieving these priorities would be played by Congress and the new administration, as the nation tries to move quickly toward national health reform. Insurance companies and state governments also have important roles. They will decide what they will pay for. Other key actors identified include the broad group of health care clinicians and researchers. And, certainly nothing will work if consumers and patients are not engaged, informed, and supported in efforts to achieve some control over their own health.

The two next steps the group identified were to catalog successful interventions and models under way around the country for both ideas and inspiration; and second, to expand and diversify the types of evidence and research used to assess integrative health care approaches.

7

Concluding Comments

First, do no harm. Then do some good.
                              —Sir Cyril Chantler

The final panel of the summit, moderated by Dr. Harvey Fineberg, allowed moderators of the five previous panels, Drs. Michael Johns, Ermina Guarneri, Bruce McEwen, Elizabeth Goldblatt, and Sean Tunis, to reflect on what they had heard during their panels and throughout the summit. This panel also provided the moderators with an opportunity to comment on what they believed were the most important issues, priorities, strategies, and unanswered questions that challenge the advancement of integrative health care.

PANEL MODERATORS
Michael M. E. Johns, Emory University

Johns began his observations by noting how summit participants had clearly articulated the need for a more coherent vision and approach to health and health care that extends over a person's lifetime. The care must pay attention to the body, the mind, and the soul and treat the individual as a full and equal partner in care decisions. Integrative health is not merely piling a series of new practitioner tools onto conventional medicine, but a whole new orientation toward person-centered care. He liked the notion that there would be an individualized plan for health over a life span. George Halvorson called this a toolkit that can integrate all health and care processes and that connects a person seamlessly with all the health care professionals.

Johns was struck by the discussion of an "optimizer" working on behalf of each individual. This could be an electronic health record or perhaps someday a telehealth application; it could be a person, serving in the role of health coach, agent, navigator, or partner; it could be a primary care provider; or it even might be a medical specialist, depending on the time, the place, and the needs of the individual. The optimizer's role would be to assure the right intervention at the right place at the right time by the right caregiver at the right value. Johns heard participants talk about the need to localize care, in the home as often as possible, and in the workplace—care should be centralized only when necessary.

Integrative health care is about healthy living, wellness, and prevention, but also, when it is needed, the proper sickness care. Johns reiterated that all these dimensions of care should be based on evidence. However, he recognized that we have to revisit the question of what evidence is and how we determine that the evidence is sufficient to recommend an intervention, therapy, or approach. This requires reinventing the evidentiary model to better assess costs and benefits, said Johns. Based on the value that specific services or approaches provide to the individual and to society, new systems of incentives and rewards can be created.

Last year, the World Health Organization reported on social and behavioral factors in health. Most Americans seem to believe such a report applies only to the developing world, Johns said. However, social determinants of health touch the lives of every American, and communities across the country struggle with poverty, education, and employment. Unless we address these social factors, all of our other efforts will not improve the health of this nation, he said.

Individuals and organizations are inevitably self-centered when it comes to their own interests, he said. This natural tendency may create significant interprofessional friction that could interfere with advancing not only integrative health care as a whole, but also the common goals that have been identified. Summit participants represented a broad mix of interests, people, backgrounds, and personalities, having notable passion, energy, and a great spirit. To ensure the success of integrative health and to overcome the potential for friction, Johns encouraged individuals and organizations to work together and harness the energy and spirit demonstrated at the summit. This may require some groups to become more selfless, and it will require all groups to embrace their unifying interests, he noted. Additional opportunities to come together may help the various professional groups to know and understand each other more deeply.

Next steps, he said, are to circulate the summary of this summit widely and to agree on language and definitions. For example, he suggested replacing *integrative medicine* with *integrative health*. Another needed step is to redefine value in health care to include not only clinical outcomes, but also patients' perceptions of their health care and its results. Finally, Johns said that stakeholders need to collaborate with patients to find a clearer, more detailed path forward—perhaps the first step should be to agree on what *health* is.

Erminia Guarneri, Scripps Center for Integrative Medicine

Guarneri noted that when she went to medical school in the 1980s she kept firmly in mind Sir William Osler's quote, "To alleviate suffering, to heal the sick, and prevent disease, this is our work." However, when her training was complete, she realized that, even for the most common and costly serious disease, her toolbox was primarily limited to a set of drugs. It did not contain anything that would have addressed the many issues covered at the summit. She was not trained in nutrition nor taught to understand that food is medicine. She was not taught that the mind can affect the physical body. What she was taught was to make a diagnosis, treat a disease, and see the next patient.

Guarneri emphasized the importance of Carol Black's inclusion of social factors in disease such as worklessness, poverty, and loneliness. The medical school curriculum typically focuses on diagnosis of disease—asthma, obesity, hypertension, diabetes. However, children raised in homes where there are rats *will* have a higher rate of asthma; children raised in poverty or with physical abuse *will* have higher rates of obesity, diabetes, and poorer overall health outcomes. Doctors can give them inhalers for the asthma, diets to follow for the obesity, and insulin for the diabetes, but if no one addresses the rats, the poverty, and the abuse, she said, these medical interventions will not be effective.

Recognizing the shortcomings in the traditional medical approach, about 13 years ago Guarneri and her team at Scripps embarked on an endeavor to prevent disease, heal people, and change lives through science and compassion. They found that a multidisciplinary team of health care providers is needed to address a disease's underlying causes, such as maladaptive responses to stress and tension, poor nutrition, and sedentary lifestyle. Now, the country is on the threshold of changing the concept of primary care, she said, and it might even be expanded to include nurse practitioners, homeopaths, naturopaths, and others. To support such an expansion requires determining the right credentials for this field of practice.

Also to be considered are ways to incentivize health care providers and employers to keep people healthy in a variety of settings, said Guarneri. The health care system, schools, workplaces, day care centers, and nursing homes should have incentives to play their part. The science on preventing many of our most serious illnesses is available, but acting on this science requires collaborative, cross-sector efforts. Guarneri said that she and the Scripps Center for Integrative Medicine are committed to improving outcomes and well-being and preventing disease, but she commented that legislation will be needed to bring a more integrative, prevention-oriented health system to fruition.

Bruce S. McEwen, Rockefeller University

McEwen reviewed the promise and challenges in developing the science base for integrative health. He said that specialization and reductionism in both medicine and science has caused the health system to lose track of the forest (whole-person health) by focusing on the trees (one body part or one system). The search for magic bullets to deal with complex, multicausation disorders has obscured the ability to appreciate, study, and manipulate the human organism as a whole, and recognize and deal effectively with the central role of the brain in regulating body systems.

Yet science already has—or can develop—tools to understand how brain and body interact. Interestingly, investigating in-depth brain function and brain–body interactions is key to understanding how even social environments affect the individual. Clinicians can work *with* the brain by altering attitudes and behavior and providing sympathetic and supportive environments, such as through the health coaches discussed at the summit, said McEwen. The science panel acknowledged the need for greater understanding of the biological foundations of thought, belief, meaning, and purpose, including ways to foster self-efficacy and self-esteem. But, he noted, people with low self-esteem may be hard to reach with messages about taking part in their own health.

Integrative health care is built on the idea of personalization. Much in current and developing science will enable this individualized care. New and better technology will help scientists measure and understand outcomes in a range of promising fields—genetic polymorphisms, epigenetics, mediators related to stress and adaptation, proteomics, telomere research, and, of course, brain function. At the same time, McEwen noted the need for sophisticated tools to make this information accessible and useful to health care practitioners and the public and for a better understanding of what it takes to motivate people to change risky behavior.

McEwen noted that basic scientists believe their research will suggest biological mechanisms that can lead to better therapies. However, they must realize that different disciplines, with different rules of evidence, will be involved in developing and implementing potential *applications* of their findings. This suggests the need to foster sustained interactions and understanding across disciplines through more interdisciplinary training and systems-oriented research. Unfortunately, young scientists interested in pursuing interdisciplinary research often confront gaps in understanding between disciplines that reduce their chances for promotion and tenure, said McEwen, and few grant reviewers have the broad knowledge and perspective necessary to assess cross-disciplinary work.

Interdisciplinary research also requires funding, noted McEwen. In the late 1990s, over the objections of many people at the National Institutes of Health, Congress authorized creation of five mind–body centers. These centers have attracted highly creative researchers who are now working on the kinds of cross-disciplinary projects that can strengthen the scientific underpinnings of integrative health care. Vigorous outreach to both policy makers and the public would help build support for continued funding of this type of research and greater application of research findings, concluded McEwen.

Elizabeth A. Goldblatt, Academic Consortium for Complementary and Alternative Health Care

To improve health and have a positive impact on lives, the social determinants of health, especially education, must be considered first, said Goldblatt. Education affects where people fit into society, their employment, and their access to health care. The poor, the unemployed, and the homeless are not thinking about diet, meditation, or yoga.

The education and workforce panelists started from the premise that the U.S. health system should shift from a disease-based to a wellness-based system that emphasizes patient-centered health care. To accomplish this, students, faculty, and practitioners not only need education within their specific fields, but they all need to be steeped in patient-centered values and in wellness, health promotion, and compassionate care. For example, they need to be taught to begin treatment with less invasive, and usually less costly, interventions before moving to more invasive ones.

Academic administrators and faculty should develop effective inter-professional education curricula and programs, she said. Students in all health disciplines could be brought together for required courses in wellness and behavior change. In this way, trainees would begin to break out of their disciplinary silos. Goldblatt reiterated that if people are educated in silos, they will practice in silos, and that style of practice is increasingly untenable. Students should also be trained to include empathy, compassion, and caring in their service to their patients.

There is a place for licensure in encouraging more multidisciplinary and interdisciplinary care teams. Licensure is valuable not only for doctors, nurses, and allied health care providers, but also for some complementary and alternative medicine practitioners—terms that Goldblatt suggests may be outdated. In describing potential participants in a person's health care team, it would be better to refer to them as licensed care providers without regard to discipline. Many of the other professional groups involved in self-care and wellness, such as yoga practitioners, meditation coaches, massage therapists, or exercise trainers, may not be required to have licenses, but many are subject to a credentialing process. Goldblatt suggested that other countries may offer insights on how best to assure the competency of such diverse team members.

U.S. health care has available superb technology and a workforce of many dedicated clinicians. However, the nation has developed a culture driven by economics that does not always support good health. High rates of obesity, diabetes, hypertension, and depression suggest that Americans are not healthy in terms of mind, body, or spirit; furthermore, she said, many Americans have lost a sense of community and mutual responsibility. For low-income Americans, there is no effective safety net, and millions are left without basic insurance coverage—something available to people in every other developed nation in the world. The stress resulting from lack of insurance, access to care, and related social support further contributes to vulnerability to illnesses. Universal health care would, she said, greatly benefit our society, culture, and the health of all Americans.

Sean Tunis, Center for Medical Technology Policy

The principal insights from the economics session, said Tunis, started with Senator Harkin's presentation, which emphasized that the United States is faced with a once-in-a-generation opportunity for major political and social change. It seems as though the economic collapse may be leading to a collapse of a culture of greed, said Tunis. There may be a greater interest in values such as internal reflection, connectedness, and community support, and these renewed values are exactly what the integrative health community focuses on. The opportunity today, both politically and socially, for the kinds of reforms that summit participants believe in, could not possibly be better, he said.

Tunis observed that the summit exposed a great deal of shared sympathy and belief in the value of integrative health care, but not much skepticism, which surprised him. He noted that not only was the level of sympathy high, but also that there was a willingness to be helpful in terms of moving things forward. There will be a lot of work to do, and this shared sympathy will be necessary to power the advancement of integrative health.

While there is clearly a great deal of evidence about the effectiveness of integrative health care and many of its component services, there is also clearly a lack of consensus about when this evidence is enough or good enough to support system reforms. In Britain, the King's Fund has done some very useful work around the evidentiary requirements for integrative health care, which may be helpful here. U.S. decision makers and policy makers will need to come to consensus on the appropriate scientific base needed.

A big part of changing the U.S. health care system would be a move from the input-based or resource-based reimbursement system to an outcome-based system, said Tunis. Such a change would be advantageous to the kinds of services and programs summit participants are committed to. However, the details will be challenging, and decisions about who is rewarded for what contribution will have to be made carefully in order to reflect what is truly meaningful in terms of health care outcomes.

Tunis's last point reiterated something several panelists mentioned, which is the importance of resisting the temptation to place blame on other sectors. Otherwise, "We will never come to any sort of constructive resolution or forward motion," said Tunis. Resisting pointing fingers is very consistent with integrative health's philosophy of respecting the individual and honoring all perspectives, he said. Finally, he predicted that integrative medicine may turn out to be the most successful approach to reforming the nation's health system.

Panel Discussion

In a concluding session, participants were asked by Fineberg to identify the most important thing they had learned throughout the course of the summit and the most important next step required to advance integrative medicine. A number of participants raised significant challenges and highlighted points from the summit presentations and discussions that were particularly salient to them.

Some participants were gratified to find out how much evidence, from diverse fields, supports the concept of integrative health care. Additional evidence that is needed could come from demonstration projects in a variety of settings, several participants said. The demonstration projects could involve examination of systems of care as well as mechanisms for health care delivery and reimbursement. Participants identified existing integrative approaches that may provide valuable information for establishing demonstration projects; one participant highlighted a Department of Defense program that includes integrative providers, and another discussed a capitated integrative medicine program offered by Blue Cross-Blue Shield of Illinois.

Several participants endorsed the idea that integrative care models should offer a wide variety of services. However, some noted that current models should give greater attention to dental care and end-of-life care, especially since a preponderance of Medicare funds is spent in the last 6 months of life. This is, in part, a result of the find-it-and-fix-it mentality, which causes patients to hope that almost anything can be fixed and causes clinicians to keep trying different treatments because they view death as a failure, suggested one participant.

Participants reiterated the need for developing and disseminating information explaining integrative care precepts to clinicians from all disciplines and to the public. One participant praised the approach used in IOM's *Crossing the Quality Chasm* report, in which an equally complex issue was translated into six succinct points. The participant noted that an analogous list could help move integrative health care forward. From the perspective of one international participant, effective promotion of the integrative health agenda and international collaboration on best approaches could help the United States learn what works in China, India, and many other nations and cultures.

A number of participants expressed support for integrative health's comprehensive, community-wide approach, and one suggested that part of what it should encompass is better control of environmental toxicities. Another suggested that efforts be made to integrate public health and environmental health at a global level.

CLOSING REMARKS
Ralph Snyderman, Duke University
Harvey V. Fineberg, Institute of Medicine

After two and a half days of informative presentations and lively discussion, Dr. Ralph Snyderman, chair of the summit planning committee, and Fineberg, President of the Institute of Medicine, thanked all of the participants for their time, their active engagement, and their energy and enthusiasm throughout the summit. Snyderman and Fineberg said the event was far bigger and far more important than the organizers could have anticipated when they began the initiative more than a year earlier.

Returning to the Rorschach blot that Fineberg discussed in his opening remarks, Snyderman reiterated that everyone had arrived at the meeting with some image of integrative medicine. However, those images were probably different in virtually every mind. Initially, he had hoped that the presentations and discussion could transform the Rorschach into the clarity of an Ansel Adams photograph that would give everyone a precise view of what integrative health care is.

While the summit did not yield a unified interpretation, many insights were attained and models presented. After hearing from so many of the participants, Snyderman was certain that almost everyone could agree that at the center of the Rorschach is an individual with unique requirements for maintaining health, preventing disease, and health care services over their lifetime. Snyderman noted that the unique individual is each of us over the course of our lives; it is our friends and family members; and it is every one of the nation's children, with their different socioeconomic backgrounds and opportunities, their different racial and ethnic identities, their different family dynamics, and their different futures.

As different as those people may be from each other and as different as their needs may be, health and well-being is a central resource to every one of them. At its root, health is about enabling people to live more fulfilling and meaningful lives. As Fineberg said, "What we are seeking most deeply in health and health care is really the same as what we are seeking in our lives."

This individual-centered approach takes into account the many components that touch lives and affect health, Snyderman noted. People are surrounded by family, friends, and larger social groups who can influence them, positively and negatively; they are exposed to various environmental factors that can help or hurt them; and with integrative health care, they can interact with a health system that can, over time, work with them to sustain health and well-being and minimize disease. Most important, if they are fortunate, they will find purpose in life and the things that are meaningful to them, to sustain them and nurture their spirit, suggested Fineberg. "For some, that feeling may arise from something as simple yet as deeply meaningful as witnessing a granddaughter's first communion, or participating in any of life's other profound moments of transition and meaning."

Snyderman observed that in the blend of discussions, there emerged a great deal of understanding, shared ideas, and inspiring hopes. He said, "The diversity of our thinking around that Rorschach, with the individual at the center and care envisioned over a lifetime, will bring us to important places. I do not know where the ideas and discussions started here will go next, but it is very important that they have started and that we all remain committed to seeing them incorporated into rational health care reform."

Snyderman noted that Fineberg was wise to ask people, near the end of the plenary session, what they had learned, what for them was different. He concluded by saying that "To some degree, all of our minds have been changed, unalterably. We are different people, capable of taking different actions. Much of what comes out of the summit will depend on the spontaneous actions and the creativity of every person in the audience. We all can play a role in keeping this movement going forward."

A

References

Anderson, G. F. 2005. Medicare and chronic conditions. *New England Journal of Medicine* 353(3):305-309.

Armaiz-Pena, G. N., S. K. Lutgendorf, S. W. Cole, and A. K. Sood. 2009. Neuroendocrine modulation of cancer progression. *Brain, Behavior, and Immunity* 23(1):10-15.

Barnes, P., B. Bloom, and R. Nahin. 2008. *National health statistics report #12. Complementary and alternative medicine use among adults and children: United States, 2007.* Hyattsville, MD: National Center for Health Statistics.

Bernhard, J. D., J. Kristeller, and J. Kabat-Zinn. 1988. Effectiveness of relaxation and visualization techniques as an adjunct to phototherapy and photochemotherapy of psoriasis. *Journal of the American Academy of Dermatology* 19(3):572-574.

Bland, J. 2008. Systems biology, functional medicine, and folates. *Alternative Therapies in Health and Medicine* 14(3):18-20.

Boden, W. E., R. A. O'Rourke, K. K. Teo, P. M. Hartigan, D. J. Maron, W. J. Kostuk, M. Knudtson, M. Dada, P. Casperson, C. L. Harris, B. R. Chaitman, L. Shaw, G. Gosselin, S. Nawaz, L. M. Title, G. Gau, A. S. Blaustein, D. C. Booth, E. R. Bates, J. A. Spertus, D. S. Berman, G. B. Mancini, and W. S. Weintraub. 2007. Optimal medical therapy with or without PCI for stable coronary disease. *New England Journal of Medicine* 356(15):1503-1516.

Burack, J. H., D. C. Barrett, R. D. Stall, M. A. Chesney, M. L. Ekstrand, and T. J. Coates. 1993. Depressive symptoms and cd4 lymphocyte decline among HIV-infected men. *Journal of the American Medical Association* 270(21):2568-2573.

Campbell, S., M. Marriott, C. Nahmias, and G. M. MacQueen. 2004. Lower hippocampal volume in patients suffering from depression: A meta-analysis. *American Journal of Psychiatry* 161(4):598-607.

Cherkas, L. F., A. Aviv, A. M. Valdes, J. L. Hunkin, J. P. Gardner, G. L. Surdulescu, M. Kimura, and T. D. Spector. 2006. The effects of social status on biological aging as measured by white-blood-cell telomere length. *Aging Cell* 5(5):361-365.

Chopra, D., D. Ornish, R. Roy, and A. Weil. 2009. "Alternative" medicine is mainstream. *Wall Street Journal*, January 9, A13.

Chou, R., and L. H. Huffman. 2007. Nonpharmacologic therapies for acute and chronic low back pain: A review of the evidence for an American Pain Society/American College of Physicians clinical practice guideline. *Annals of Internal Medicine* 147(7):492-504.

Christensen, C. M., J. H. Grossman, and J. Hwang. 2009. *The innovator's prescription: A disruptive solution for health care.* New York: McGraw-Hill.

Cizza, G., A. H. Marques, F. Eskandari, I. C. Christie, S. Torvik, M. N. Silverman, T. M. Phillips, and E. M. Sternberg. 2008. Elevated neuroimmune biomarkers in sweat patches and plasma of premenopausal women with major depressive disorder in remission: The power study. *Biological Psychiatry* 64(10):907-911.

Cochrane, A. L. 1999. *Effectiveness and efficiency: Random reflections on health services,* 2nd ed. London, UK: Royal Society of Medicine Press.

Cohen, S., W. J. Doyle, D. P. Skoner, B. S. Rabin, and J. M. Gwaltney, Jr. 1997. Social ties and susceptibility to the common cold. *Journal of the American Medical Association* 277(24):1940-1944.

Cohen, S., D. Janicki-Deverts, and G. E. Miller. 2007. Psychological stress and disease. *Journal of the American Medical Association* 298(14):1685-1687.

Conrad, C. D. 2006. What is the functional significance of chronic stress-induced ca3 dendritic retraction within the hippocampus? *Behavioral and Cognitive Neuroscience Reviews* 5(1):41-60.

Cooper, R. A., T. E. Getzen, H. J. McKee, and P. Laud. 2002. Economic and demographic trends signal an impending physician shortage. *Health Affairs* 21(1):140-154.

de Lange, F. P., A. Koers, J. S. Kalkman, G. Bleijenberg, P. Hagoort, J. W. van der Meer, and I. Toni. 2008. Increase in prefrontal cortical volume following cognitive behavioural therapy in patients with chronic fatigue syndrome. *Brain* 131(Pt 8):2172-2180.

Dolinoy, D. C., J. R. Weidman, R. A. Waterland, and R. L. Jirtle. 2006. Maternal genistein alters coat color and protects Avy mouse offspring from obesity by modifying the fetal epigenome. *Environmental Health Perspectives* 114(4):567-572.

Dolinoy, D. C., D. Huang, and R. L. Jirtle. 2007. Maternal nutrient supplementation counteracts bisphenol A-induced DNA hypomethylation in early development. *Proceedings of the National Academy of Sciences of the United States of America* 104(32):13056-13061.

Druss, B. G., S. C. Marcus, M. Olfson, T. Tanielian, L. Elinson, and H. A. Pincus. 2001. Comparing the national economic burden of five chronic conditions. *Health Affairs* 20(6):233-241.

Dusek, J. A., P. L. Hibberd, B. Buczynski, B. H. Chang, K. C. Dusek, J. M. Johnston, A. L. Wohlhueter, H. Benson, and R. M. Zusman. 2008. Stress management versus lifestyle modification on systolic hypertension and medication elimination: A randomized trial. *Journal of Alternative and Complementary Medicine* 14(2):129-138.

Epel, E. S., E. H. Blackburn, J. Lin, F. S. Dhabhar, N. E. Adler, J. D. Morrow, and R. M. Cawthon. 2004. Accelerated telomere shortening in response to life stress. *Proceedings of the National Academy of Sciences of the United States of America* 101(49):17312-17315.

Erickson, K. I., and A. F. Kramer. 2009. Aerobic exercise effects on cognitive and neural plasticity in older adults. *British Journal of Sports Medicine* 43(1):22-24.

Flexner, A. 1910. *Medical education in the United States and Canada: A report to the Carnegie Foundation for the Advancement of Teaching.* New York: Carnegie Foundation for the Advancement of Teaching.

Forster, A. J., H. J. Murff, J. F. Peterson, T. K. Gandhi, and D. W. Bates. 2003. The incidence and severity of adverse events affecting patients after discharge from the hospital. *Annals of Internal Medicine* 138(3):161-167.

Frasure-Smith, N., F. Lesperance, and M. Talajic. 1993. Depression following myocardial infarction. Impact on 6-month survival. *Journal of the American Medical Association* 270(15):1819-1825.

GAO (Government Accountability Office). 2008. *Primary care professionals: Recent trends, projections, and valuation of services.* Washington, DC: GAO.

Gould, K. L., D. Ornish, L. Scherwitz, S. Brown, R. P. Edens, M. J. Hess, N. Mullani, L. Bolomey, F. Dobbs, W. T. Armstrong, T. Merritt, T. Ports, S. Sparler, and J. Billings. 1995. Changes in myocardial perfusion abnormalities by positron emission tomography after long-term, intense risk factor modification. *Journal of the American Medical Association* 274(11):894-901.

Haake, M., H. H. Muller, C. Schade-Brittinger, H. D. Basler, H. Schafer, C. Maier, H. G. Endres, H. J. Trampisch, and A. Molsberger. 2007. German acupuncture trials (GERAC) for chronic low back pain: Randomized, multicenter, blinded, parallel-group trial with 3 groups. *Archives of Internal Medicine* 167(17):1892-1898.

Hope, T. 1997. Evidence-based patient choice and the doctor-patient relationship. In *But will it work, doctor?* London: Kings Fund.

Hyman, M. 2007. Systems biology, toxins, obesity, and functional medicine. *Alternative Therapies in Health and Medicine* 13(2):S134-S139.

IOM (Institute of Medicine). 1999. *To err is human: Building a safer health system.* Washington, DC: National Academy Press.

IOM. 2001a. *Crossing the quality chasm: A new health system for the 21st century.* Washington, DC: National Academy Press.

IOM. 2001b. *Health and Behavior: The Interplay of Biological, Behavioral, and Societal Influences.* Washington, DC: National Academy Press.

IOM. 2005. *From Cancer Patient to Cancer Survivor: Lost in Transition.* Washington, DC: The National Academies Press.

IOM. 2007a. *Ending the Tobacco Problem: A Blueprint for the Nation.* Washington, DC: The National Academies Press.

IOM. 2007b. *Rewarding provider performance: Aligning incentives in Medicare.* Washington, DC: The National Academies Press.

IOM. 2008. *Cancer Care for the Whole Patient: Meeting Psychosocial Health Needs.* Washington, DC: The National Academies Press.

Jonsen, A. R. 1990. *The new medicine and the old ethics.* Boston, MA: Harvard University Press.

Keehan, S., A. Sisko, C. Truffer, S. Smith, C. Cowan, J. Poisal, M. K. Clemens, and the National Health Expenditure Accounts Projections Team. 2008. Health spending projections through 2017: The baby-boom generation is coming to Medicare. *Health Affairs* 27(2):w145-w155.

Kiecolt-Glaser, J. K., P. T. Marucha, W. B. Malarkey, A. M. Mercado, and R. Glaser. 1995. Slowing of wound healing by psychological stress. *Lancet* 346(8984):1194-1196.

King, M. C., J. H. Marks, and J. B. Mandell. 2003. Breast and ovarian cancer risks due to inherited mutations in BRCA1 and BRCA2. *Science* 302(5645):643-646.

Knowler, W. C., E. Barrett-Connor, S. E. Fowler, R. F. Hamman, J. M. Lachin, E. A. Walker, and D. M. Nathan. 2002. Reduction in the incidence of type 2 diabetes with lifestyle intervention or metformin. *New England Journal of Medicine* 346(6):393-403.

Lantz, P. M., J. S. House, J. M. Lepkowski, D. R. Williams, R. P. Mero, and J. Chen. 1998. Socioeconomic factors, health behaviors, and mortality: Results from a nationally representative prospective study of us adults. *Journal of the American Medical Association* 279(21):1703-1708.

Mare, R. D. 1990. Socio-economic careers and differential mortality among older men in the U.S. In *Measurement and analysis of mortality—new approaches*, edited by J. Vallin, S. D'Souza and A. Palloni. Clarendon, UK: Oxford. Pp. 362-387.

Marmot, M. 2004. *The status syndrome: How social status affects our health and longevity*. New York: Times Books.

Mayne, T. J., E. Vittinghoff, M. A. Chesney, D. C. Barrett, and T. J. Coates. 1996. Depressive affect and survival among gay and bisexual men infected with HIV. *Archives of Internal Medicine* 156(19):2233-2238.

McEwen, B. S. 1998. Protective and damaging effects of stress mediators. *New England Journal of Medicine* 338(3):171-179.

McGlynn, E. A., S. M. Asch, J. Adams, J. Keesey, J. Hicks, A. DeCristofaro, and E. A. Kerr. 2003. The quality of health care delivered to adults in the United States. *New England Journal of Medicine* 348(26):2635-2645.

Mechanic, D., L. B. Rogut, D. Colby, and J. R. Knickman, eds. 2005. *Policy challenges in modern health care*. New Brunswick, NJ: Rutgers University Press.

Nahin, R.L., P.M. Barnes, B.J. Stussman, and B. Bloom. *National health statistics report #18. Costs of Complementary and Alternative Medicine (CAM) and Frequency of Visits to CAM Practitioners: United States, 2007.* Hyattsville, MD: National Center for Health Statistics. 2009.

National Business Group on Health. 2007. *A purchaser's guide to clinical preventive services: Moving science into coverage*. Washington, DC: National Business Group on Health.

National Health Service Institute for Innovation and Improvement. 2009. *Working with others*. http://www.institute.nhs.uk/assessment_tool/general/working_with_others.html (accessed May 19, 2009).

National Institutes of Health. 2006. State-of-the-science conference statement: Multivitamin/mineral supplements and chronic disease prevention. *Annals of Internal Medicine* 145(5):364-371.

Nerem, R. M., M. J. Levesque, and J. F. Cornhill. 1980. Social environment as a factor in diet-induced atherosclerosis. *Science* 208 (4451):1475-1476.

Newton, B. W., L. Barber, J. Clardy, E. Cleveland, and P. O'Sullivan. 2008. Is there hardening of the heart during medical school? *Academic Medicine* 83(3):244-249.

OECD (Organisation for Economic Co-operation and Development). 2009. *Society at a glance 2009—OECD social indicators.* Paris, France: OECD.

Ornish, D. 2009. *Persistence with statin therapy (source: National Drug Code Health Information Services, 1998), in the Science of Integrative Medicine.* Speech at IOM Summit on Integrative Medicine and the Health of the Public, Washington, DC, February 26.

Ornish, D., A. M. Gotto, and R. R. Miller, et al. 1979. Effects of a vegetarian diet and selected yoga techniques in the treatment of coronary heart disease. *Clinical Research* 27:720A.

Ornish, D., L. W. Scherwitz, R. S. Doody, D. Kesten, S. M. McLanahan, S. E. Brown, E. DePuey, R. Sonnemaker, C. Haynes, J. Lester, G. K. McAllister, R. J. Hall, J. A. Burdine, and A. M. Gotto, Jr. 1983. Effects of stress management training and dietary changes in treating ischemic heart disease. *Journal of the American Medical Association* 249(1):54-59.

Ornish, D., S. E. Brown, L. W. Scherwitz, J. H. Billings, W. T. Armstrong, T. A. Ports, S. M. McLanahan, R. L. Kirkeeide, R. J. Brand, and K. L. Gould. 1990. Can lifestyle changes reverse coronary heart disease? The lifestyle heart trial. *Lancet* 336(8708):129-133.

Ornish, D., L. W. Scherwitz, J. H. Billings, S. E. Brown, K. L. Gould, T. A. Merritt, S. Sparler, W. T. Armstrong, T. A. Ports, R. L. Kirkeeide, C. Hogeboom, and R. J. Brand. 1998. Intensive lifestyle changes for reversal of coronary heart disease. *Journal of the American Medical Association* 280(23):2001-2007.

Ornish, D., G. Weidner, W. R. Fair, R. Marlin, E. B. Pettengill, C. J. Raisin, S. Dunn-Emke, L. Crutchfield, F. N. Jacobs, R. J. Barnard, W. J. Aronson, P. McCormac, D. J. McKnight, J. D. Fein, A. M. Dnistrian, J. Weinstein, T. H. Ngo, N. R. Mendell, and P. R. Carroll. 2005. Intensive lifestyle changes may affect the progression of prostate cancer. *Journal of Urology* 174(3):1065-1069; discussion 1069-1070.

Ornish, D., M. J. Magbanua, G. Weidner, V. Weinberg, C. Kemp, C. Green, M. D. Mattie, R. Marlin, J. Simko, K. Shinohara, C. M. Haqq, and P. R. Carroll. 2008a. Changes in prostate gene expression in men undergoing an intensive nutrition and lifestyle intervention. *Proceedings of the National Academy of Sciences of the United States of America* 105(24):8369-8374.

Ornish, D., J. Lin, J. Daubenmier, G. Weidner, E. Epel, C. Kemp, M. J. Magbanua, R. Marlin, L. Yglecias, P. R. Carroll, and E. H. Blackburn. 2008b. Increased telomerase activity and comprehensive lifestyle changes: A pilot study. *Lancet Oncology* 9(11):1048-1057.

Page, S. J., P. Levine, and A. Leonard. 2007. Mental practice in chronic stroke: Results of a randomized, placebo-controlled trial. *Stroke* 38(4):1293-1297.

Pamuk, E., D. Makuc, K. Heck, C. Reuben, and K. Lochner. 1998. Health, United States, 1998. In *Socioeconomic status and health chartbook*. Hyattsville, MD: National Center for Health Statistics. Pp. 145-159.

Pappas, G., S. Queen, W. Hadden, and G. Fisher. 1993. The increasing disparity in mortality between socioeconomic groups in the United States, 1960 and 1986. *New England Journal of Medicine* 329(2):103-109.

Pelletier, K. R. 2009 (in press). A review and assessment of clinical and cost outcomes of comprehensive health promotion and disease management programs in the worksite: Update vii: 2004-2008. *Journal of Occupational and Environmental Medicine*.

Pelletier, K. R., P. M. Herman, R. D. Metz, and C. F. Nelson. Unpublished. *Health and medical economics: Applications to integrative medicine*. Walnut Creek, CA: University of Arizona and University of California (UCSF) Schools of Medicine.

Prochaska, J. O., and C. C. DiClemente. 1983. Stages and processes of self-change of smoking: Toward an integrative model of change. *Journal of Consulting and Clinical Psychology* 51(3):390-395.

Reeves, S., M. Zwarenstein, J. Goldman, H. Barr, D. Freeth, M. Hammick, and I. Koppel. 2008. Interprofessional education: Effects on professional practice and health care outcomes. *Cochrane Database of Systematic Reviews 2008*(1):CD002213. DOI: 002210.001002/14651858.CD14002213.pub14651852.

Reik, W., W. Dean, and J. Walter. 2001. Epigenetic reprogramming in mammalian development. *Science* 293(5532):1089-1093.

Repetti, R. L., S. E. Taylor, and T. E. Seeman. 2002. Risky families: Family social environments and the mental and physical health of offspring. *Psychological Bulletin* 128(2):330-366.

Robert Wood Johnson Foundation. 2008. *Overcoming obstacles to health.* Princeton, NJ: Robert Wood Johnson Foundation.

Schoen, C., K. Davis, S. K. H. How, and S. C. Schoenbaum. 2006. U.S. Health system performance: A national scorecard. *Health Affairs* 25(6):w457-w475.

Sheline, Y. I., M. H. Gado, and H. C. Kraemer. 2003. Untreated depression and hippocampal volume loss. *American Journal of Psychiatry* 160(8):1516-1518.

Sherman, K. J., D. C. Cherkin, J. Erro, D. L. Miglioretti, and R. A. Deyo. 2005. Comparing yoga, exercise, and a self-care book for chronic low back pain: A randomized, controlled trial. *Annals of Internal Medicine* 143(12):849-856.

Shoba, G., D. Joy, T. Joseph, M. Majeed, R. Rajendran, and P. S. Srinivas. 1998. Influence of piperine on the pharmacokinetics of curcumin in animals and human volunteers. *Planta Medica* 64(4):353-356.

Slade, S. C., and J. L. Keating. 2007. Unloaded movement facilitation exercise compared to no exercise or alternative therapy on outcomes for people with nonspecific chronic low back pain: A systematic review. *Journal of Manipulative and Physiological Therapeutics* 30(4):301-311.

Snyderman, R., and R. S. Williams. 2003. Prospective medicine: The next health care transformation. *Academic Medicine* 78(11):1079-1084.

Spiegel, D., J. R. Bloom, H. C. Kraemer, and E. Gottheil. 1989. Effect of psychosocial treatment on survival of patients with metastatic breast cancer. *Lancet* 2(8668):888-891.

Spiegel, D., L. D. Butler, J. Giese-Davis, C. Koopman, E. Miller, S. DiMiceli, C. C. Classen, P. Fobair, R. W. Carlson, and H. C. Kraemer. 2007. Effects of supportive-expressive group therapy on survival of patients with metastatic breast cancer: A randomized prospective trial. *Cancer* 110(5):1130-1138.

U.S. Congress, Senate Committee on Finance. 2006. *Testimony of Paul H. O'Neill.* 109th Congress, 2nd Session. March 8.

U.S. Congress, Senate Health, Education, Labor, and Pension Committee. 2004. *Testimony of Arnold Milstein.* 108th Congress, 2nd Session. January 28,.

van Helden, Y. G., J. Keijer, A. M. Knaapen, S. G. Heil, J. J. Briede, F. J. van Schooten, and R. W. Godschalk. 2009. Beta-carotene metabolites enhance inflammation-induced oxidative DNA damage in lung epithelial cells. *Free Radical Biology and Medicine* 46(2):299-304.

Waddell, G., and A. K. Burton. 2006. *Is work good for your health and well being?* London: The Stationery Office.

Waterland, R. A., and R. L. Jirtle. 2003. Transposable elements: Targets for early nutritional effects on epigenetic gene regulation. *Molecular and Cellular Biology* 23(15):5293-5300.

Weston, A. D., and L. Hood. 2004. Systems biology, proteomics, and the future of health care: Toward predictive, preventative, and personalized medicine. *Journal of Proteome Research* 3(2):179-196.

Yusuf, S., S. Hawken, S. Ounpuu, T. Dans, A. Avezum, F. Lanas, M. McQueen, A. Budaj, P. Pais, J. Varigos, and L. Lisheng. 2004. Effect of potentially modifiable risk factors associated with myocardial infarction in 52 countries (the INTERHEART study): Case-control study. *Lancet* 364(9438):937-952.

B

Meeting Agenda

Summit on Integrative Medicine
and the Health of the Public

FEBRUARY 25–27, 2009
NATIONAL ACADEMY OF SCIENCES BUILDING
WASHINGTON, DC

DAY ONE (February 25)

9:00 a.m.   **Welcome and opening remarks**
Harvey Fineberg, Institute of Medicine

9:15   **Keynote I. Stage setting: Integrating health and health care**
Ralph Snyderman, Duke University

10:00   **BREAK**

10:15   **Panel I. Vision: What is needed for an integrative approach to health?**
Panel moderator: *Michael Johns, Emory University*
- *William Novelli, AARP*
- *George Halvorson, Kaiser Permanente*
- *Victor Sierpina, University of Texas Medical Branch*
- *Ellen Stovall, National Coalition for Cancer Survivorship*
- *Mehmet Oz, New York-Presbyterian Hospital/Columbia University Medical Center*

175

11:45   **LUNCH AND DISCUSSION SESSIONS**

Health care reform agenda (Lecture Room)
Discussion leaders:
- *Lawrence Lewin, Executive Consultant*
- *Arnold Milstein, Pacific Business Group on Health*

Economic realities of integrative medicine (Members Room)
Discussion leaders:
- *Kenneth Pelletier, University of Arizona and University of California (UCSF) Schools of Medicine*
- *Marcel Salive, Center for Medicare and Medicaid Services*

Evaluating the evidence base (Board Room)
Discussion leaders:
- *Kenneth Brigham, Emory University*
- *Bruce McEwen, Rockefeller University*
- *Josephine Briggs, NIH National Center for Complementary and Alternative Medicine*
- *Larry Green, University of California, San Francisco*

Education/workforce of integrative medicine (Room 150)
Discussion leaders:
- *Cyril Chantler, King's Fund*
- *Aviad Haramati, Georgetown University School of Medicine*
- *Victor Sierpina, University of Texas Medical Branch*

1:15 p.m.   **Priority assessment group reports**
Moderator: *Ralph Snyderman, Duke University*
Rapporteurs:
- *Reed Tuckson, UnitedHealth*
- *Fred Sanfilippo, Emory Healthcare*

2:15   **Panel II. The models**
            Panel moderator: *Erminia Guarneri, Scripps Center*
            for Integrative Medicine
            ▪ *Models to ensure integrated, continuous care,*
                including chronic disease across caregivers and
                settings
                – *Edward Wagner, MacColl Institute for*
                    Healthcare Innovation at Group Health Center
                    for Health Studies
            ▪ *Care models to lower near-term per capita spending*
                responsibly
                – *Arnold Milstein, Mercer*
            ▪ *Models to promote health and wellness, prevention,*
                management of chronic diseases
                – *David Katz, Yale University*
            ▪ *Models to optimize health and healing across the*
                lifespan
                – *Tracy Gaudet, Duke University*
            ▪ *Models to promote primary care (medical home,*
                patient-centered care)
                – *Mike Magee, Center for Aging Services*
                    Technologies

3:45   **BREAK**

4:00   **Keynote II. The models**
            Donald Berwick, Institute for Healthcare Improvement

4:45   **ADJOURN**

            DAY TWO (February 26)

9:00 a.m.   **Keynote III. The science**
            Dean Ornish, Preventive Medicine Research Institute

9:45   **Panel III. The science**
            Panel moderator: *Bruce McEwen, Rockefeller*
            University
            ▪ *Social determinants of health*
                – *Nancy Adler, University of California, San*
                    Francisco

- *Mind–body medicine*
  - *Esther Sternberg, NIH National Institute of Mental Health*
- *Genomic/predictive medicine*
  - *Richard Lifton, Yale University*
- *Environmental epigenetics*
  - *Mitchell Gaynor, Weill-Cornell Medical Center and Gaynor Integrative Oncology*
- *Intervention evaluation and outcomes measures*
  - *Lawrence Green, University of California, San Francisco*
- *CAM modalities*
  - *Josephine Briggs, NIH National Center for Complementary and Alternative Medicine*

11:30   **LUNCH AND DISCUSSION SESSIONS**

Enhancing wellness (Lecture Room)
Discussion leaders:
- *Jon Kabat-Zinn, Center for Mindfulness in Medicine*
- *William George, Harvard Business School*

Mind–body–societal connections (Members Room)
Discussion Leaders:
- *Esther Sternberg, National Institutes of Health*
- *James Gordon, Center for Mind-Body Medicine*

Models of integrative medicine (Board Room)
Discussion Leaders:
- *Mike Magee, Center for Aging Services Technologies*
- *Tracy Gaudet, Duke Integrative Medicine*

Public perspective of integrative medicine (Room 150)
Discussion Leaders:
- *Ellen Stovall, National Coalition for Cancer Survivorship*
- *Judy Miller Jones, National Health Policy Forum*
- *Mary Woolley, Research! America*

1:00 p.m.   **Priority assessment group reports**
            Moderator: *Ralph Snyderman, Duke University*
            Rapporteurs:
            - *Richard Lifton, Yale University*
            - *Aviad Haramati, Georgetown University*
            - *Helen Darling, National Business Group on Health*

2:00   **Panel IV. Workforce and education**
            Panel moderator: *Elizabeth Goldblatt, Council of*
            Colleges of Acupuncture and Oriental Medicine
            - *Education curricula*
              - *Mary Jo Kreitzer, University of Minnesota*
            - *Core competencies*
              - *Victoria Maizes, University of Arizona*
            - *Interprofessional education*
              - *Adam Perlman, University of Medicine &*
                Dentistry of New Jersey
            - *Workforce reorientation*
              - *Richard Cooper, University of Pennsylvania*
            - *Standards, regulation, and patient safety*
              - *Cyril Chantler, King's Fund*

3:30   **BREAK**

3:45   **Keynote IV. Workforce and education**
            Carol Black, Academy of Medical Royal Colleges

4:30   **ADJOURN**

            DAY THREE (February 27)

8:30 a.m.   **Keynote V. The economics**
            Senator Tom Harkin, U.S. Senate

9:15   **Panel V. The economics**
            Panel moderator: *Sean Tunis, Center for Medical*
            Technology Policy
            - *Economic burden of chronic disease*
            Kenneth Thorpe, Emory University
            - *Insurer perspective*
              - *Reed Tuckson, UnitedHealth Group*

- *Employer perspective*
  - *Tom Donohue, U.S. Chamber of Commerce*
  - *William George, Harvard University*
- *Behavior change incentives and approaches*
  - *Janet Kahn, University of Vermont*
- *Rewards of integrative medicine*
  - *Kenneth Pelletier, University of Arizona and University of California (UCSF) Schools of Medicine*

10:45 **BREAK**

11:00 **Panel VI. Issues, priorities, and strategies: Moving forward**
Panel moderator: *Harvey Fineberg, Institute of Medicine*
Panelists: Moderators from previous panels
- *Michael Johns, Emory University*
- *Erminia Guarneri, Scripps Center for Integrative Medicine*
- *Bruce McEwen, Rockefeller University*
- *Elizabeth Goldblatt, Council of Colleges of Acupuncture and Oriental Medicine*
- *Sean Tunis, Center for Medical Technology Policy*

12:20 p.m. **Final remarks**
Ralph Snyderman, Duke University
Harvey Fineberg, Institute of Medicine

12:30 **ADJOURN**

PLANNING COMMITTEE

Ralph Snyderman (Chair), Duke University
Carol M. Black, Academy of Medical Royal Colleges
Cyril Chantler, The King's Fund
Erminia Guarneri, Scripps Center for Integrative
  Medicine
Elizabeth A. Goldblatt, Academic Consortium for
  Complementary and Alternative Health Care
Richard P. Lifton, Yale University
Michael M. E. Johns, Emory University
Bruce S. McEwen, Rockefeller University
Dean Ornish, Preventive Medicine Research Institute and
  University of California, San Francisco
Victor S. Sierpina, University of Texas Medical Branch
Esther M. Sternberg, NIH National Institute of Mental
  Health
Ellen L. Stovall, National Coalition for Cancer Survivorship
Reed V. Tuckson, UnitedHealth Group
Sean Tunis, Center for Medical Technology Policy

C

Priority Assessment Group Participants and Luncheon Discussion Leaders

PRIORITY ASSESSMENT GROUP PARTICIPANTS

February 25, 2009

Integrative medicine and its role in shaping the national health reform agenda

Moderator: Elizabeth Goldblatt, American College of Traditional Chinese Medicine

Rapporteur: Reed Tuckson, UnitedHealth

Susan Bauer-Wu, Emory University

Jeffrey Bland, Metagenics, Inc.

Sherman Cohn, Georgetown University

Simon Fielding, Foundation for Integrated Health

Susan Folkman, Osher Center for Integrative Medicine

Christy Mack, The Bravewell Collaborative

Diane Neimann, The Bravewell Collaborative

Margaret O'Kane, National Committee for Quality Assurance

Badri Rickhi, Canadian Institute of Natural and Integrative Medicine

Identifying and advancing workable models of care

Moderator: Carol Black, Academy of Medical Royal Colleges

Rapporteur: Fred Sanfilippo, Emory Healthcare

Brian Berman, University of Maryland

Lilian Cheung, Harvard University

Mary Hardy, Venice Free Clinic

Mark Hyman, Institute for Functional Medicine

Bradly Jacobs, University of California, San Francisco

183

Woodson Merrell, Albert Einstein School of Medicine
Charles Sawyer, Northwestern Health Sciences University
Timothy Birdsall, Cancer Treatment Centers of America
Lori Knutson, Penny George Institute for Health and Healing

February 26, 2009

Advancing the science base
Moderator: Bruce McEwen, Rockefeller University
Rapporteur: Richard Lifton, Yale University
Donald Abrams, Osher Center for Integrative Medicine
Kenneth Brigham, Emory University
Margaret Chesney, University of Maryland
Gary Deng, Memorial Sloan-Kettering Cancer Center
Wayne Jonas, Samueli Institute
Lixing Lao, University of Maryland
Patrick Mansky, NIH National Center for Complementary and
    Alternative Medicine
Rustum Roy, Pennsylvania State University
Alan Trachtenberg, Indian Health Service

Reorienting the workforce
Moderator: Victor Sierpina, University of Texas Medical Branch
Rapporteur: Aviad Haramati, Georgetown University
Adam Burke, San Francisco State University
Lee Chin, Dana-Farber/Brigham and Women's Cancer Center
Timothy Culbert, University of Minnesota
Patrick Hanaway, American Board of Integrative Holistic Medicine
Mary Jo Kreitzer, University of Minnesota
Roberta Lee, Department of Integrative Medicine at Beth Israel Medical
    Center
Karen Malone, University of Medicine and Dentistry of New Jersey
William Meeker, Palmer Center for Chiropractic Research
David Rakel, University of Wisconsin

Designing and building the economic incentives
Moderator: Sean Tunis, Center for Medical Technology Policy
Rapporteur: Helen Darling, National Business Group on Health
Eric Caplan, Lewin Group

Robert DeNoble, Marino Center for Integrative Health
Erminia Guarneri, Scripps Center for Integrative Medicine
Patricia Herman, University of Arizona
Davis Masten, Cheskin and the National Academies Presidents' Circle
Anne Nedrow, Consortium of Academic Health Centers for Integrative
    Medicine/Oregon Health Sciences University
William Rollow, Enhanced Care Initiatives
Richard Sarnat, AMI Groups
Michelle Simon, Seattle Healing Arts Center

LUNCHEON DISCUSSION LEADERS

February 25, 2009

Health care reform agenda
Lawrence Lewin, Executive Consultant
Arnold Milstein, Pacific Business Group on Health

Economic realities of integrative medicine
Kenneth Pelletier, University of Arizona and University of California
    (UCSF) Schools of Medicine
Marcel Salive, Center for Medicare and Medicaid Services

Evaluating the evidence base
Kenneth Brigham, Emory University
Bruce McEwen, Rockefeller University
Josephine Briggs, NIH National Center for Complementary and
    Alternative Medicine
Lawrence Green, University of California, San Francisco

Education/workforce of integrative medicine
Cyril Chantler, King's Fund
Aviad Haramati, Georgetown University School of Medicine
Victor Sierpina, University of Texas Medical Branch

February 26, 2009

Enhancing wellness
Jon Kabat-Zinn, Center for Mindfulness in Medicine
William George, Harvard Business School

Mind–body–societal connections
Esther Sternberg, National Institutes of Health
James Gordon, Center for Mind-Body Medicine

Models of integrative medicine
Mike Magee, Center for Aging Services Technologies
Tracy Gaudet, Duke Integrative Medicine

Public perspective of integrative medicine
Ellen Stovall, National Coalition for Cancer Survivorship
Judy Miller Jones, National Health Policy Forum
Mary Woolley, Research! America

D

Speaker and Staff Biographies

SPEAKER BIOGRAPHIES

Nancy E. Adler, Ph.D.
Dr. Adler is Professor of Psychology, Departments of Psychiatry and Pediatrics at the University of California, San Francisco, where she is also Vice Chair of the Department of Psychiatry, and Director of the Center for Health and Community. Dr. Adler is a Fellow of the American Psychological Society and the American Psychological Association. She is a member of the Society for Experimental Social Psychology, the Academy of Behavioral Medicine Research, the Society for Behavioral Medicine, and the Institute of Medicine. Dr. Adler's earlier research examined the utility of decision models for understanding health behaviors with particular focus on reproductive health. This work identified both determinants and consequences of unwanted pregnancy. Her current work examines the pathways from socioeconomic status (SES) to health. As Director of the MacArthur Foundation Research Network on SES and Health, she coordinates research spanning social, psychological, and biological mechanisms by which SES influences health.

Donald M. Berwick, M.D., M.P.P., FRCP
Dr. Berwick is President and CEO of the Institute for Healthcare Improvement. He is one of the nation's leading authorities on health care quality and improvement issues. He is also Clinical Professor of Pediatrics and Health Care Policy at the Harvard Medical School. Dr. Berwick has served as Vice Chair of the U.S. Preventive Services Task Force, the first Independent Member of the Board of Trustees of the American Hospital Association, and as Chair on the National Advisory Council of

the Agency for Healthcare Research and Quality. He served on President Clinton's Advisory Commission on Consumer Protection and Quality in the Healthcare Industry. Co-chaired by the Secretaries of Health and Human Services and Labor, the commission was charged with developing a broader understanding of issues facing the rapidly evolving health care delivery system and building consensus on ways to assure and improve the quality of health care.

Carol Black, D.B.E., M.D., FRCP, FMedSci
(planning committee member)
Professor Dame Carol Black is the National Director for Health and Work, Chairman of the Nuffield Trust, and Chairman of the Academy of Medical Royal Colleges. Her unit at the Royal Free Hospital, London, is the major center in Europe for clinical care and research on systemic sclerosis and is internationally renowned. Since the mid-1990s, she has worked at board level in a number of organizations: the Royal College of Physicians, the Royal Free Hospital Hampstead National Health Service (NHS) Trust, the Health Foundation, the NHS Institute for Innovation and Improvement, and St. Mary's and Hammersmith Hospitals Charitable Funds. She is also a member of many national committees aiming to improve health care. She is a Foreign Affiliate of the Institute of Medicine and has been awarded many honorary degrees and fellowships.

Josephine P. Briggs, M.D.
Dr. Briggs was named Director of the National Center for Complementary and Alternative Medicine on January 24, 2008. An accomplished researcher and physician, Dr. Briggs brings a focus on translational research to the study of complementary and alternative medicine (CAM) to help build a fuller understanding of the usefulness and safety of CAM practices. Dr. Briggs joined the National Institutes of Health (NIH) in 1997 as Director of the Division of Kidney, Urologic, and Hematologic Diseases at the National Institute of Diabetes and Digestive and Kidney Diseases (NIDDK) where she oversaw extramural research activities in kidney and urological disease. While at NIDDK, she cochaired an NIH Roadmap Committee on Translational Core Resources. From 2006 to 2008, she served as Senior Scientific Officer at the Howard Hughes Medical Institute. Dr. Briggs' research interests include the renin-angiotensin system, diabetic nephropathy, circadian regulation of blood pressure, and the effect of antioxidants in kidney disease.

Cyril Chantler
(planning committee member)
Cyril Chantler is Chairman of the King's Fund, London, and of University College London Partners. He is Chairman of the Beit Memorial Fellowships Board. He is a trustee of the Dunhill Medical Trust, a member of the Council of Southwark Cathedral, and a member of the editorial board of the *Journal of the American Medical Association*. Cyril Chantler was Dean of the Guy's, King's College and St. Thomas' Hospitals' Medical and Dental School, where he was the Children Nationwide Medical Research Fund Professor of Pediatric Nephrology until his retirement in 2000. Previously, he was Principal of the United Medical and Dental School of Guy's and St. Thomas's Hospitals (1992 to 1998) and General Manager of Guy's Hospital (1985 to 1988). He was Chairman of Great Ormond Street Hospital for Children (2001 to 2008) and of the Clinical Advisory Group for National Health Service London (2007 to 2008).

Richard A. Cooper, M.D.
Dr. Cooper is a Professor of Medicine and Senior Fellow in the Leonard Davis Institute of Health Economics at the University of Pennsylvania. Following 2 years on the faculty at Harvard, Dr. Cooper became Chief of the Hematology Section in the Department of Medicine of the University of Pennsylvania and subsequently Director of Penn's Cancer Center, positions he held for 14 years. In 1985 he moved to the Medical College of Wisconsin in Milwaukee, where he served as Executive Vice President and Dean and subsequently as the Director of the College's Health Policy Institute. In 2005, he returned to the University of Pennsylvania as a Professor of Medicine in the Leonard Davis Institute of Health Economics. Over the past 15 years, Dr. Cooper has focused on issues related to the supply of physicians and nonphysician clinicians, including the development of the Trend Model for estimating future demand and the Affluence–Poverty Nexus, a multidimensional framework that explains geographic variation in health care resources and utilization.

Thomas J. Donohue
Thomas J. Donohue is President and CEO of the U.S. Chamber of Commerce. Since assuming his position in 1997, Donohue has built the Chamber into a lobbying and political force with expanded influence across the globe. Under Donohue's leadership, the Chamber has emerged as a major player in election politics, and it has tripled its annual reve-

nues to more than $130 million. Prior to his current post, Donohue served for 13 years as President and CEO of the American Trucking Associations, the national organization of the trucking industry. Donohue is President of the Center for International Private Enterprise, a program of the National Endowment for Democracy dedicated to the development of market-oriented institutions around the world. Born in New York City in 1938, Donohue earned a bachelor's degree from St. John's University and a master's degree in business administration from Adelphi University.

Harvey V. Fineberg, M.D., Ph.D.
Dr. Fineberg is President of the Institute of Medicine. He previously served Harvard University as Provost and as Dean of the School of Public Health. He also has served as President of the Society for Medical Decision Making and Consultant to the World Health Organization. His research has included assessment of medical technology, evaluation of vaccines, and dissemination of medical innovations. He is the author or coauthor of numerous books and articles on subjects ranging from AIDS prevention to medical education. Fineberg holds four degrees from Harvard, including the M.D. and Ph.D. in Public Policy.

Tracy Gaudet, M.D.
Dr. Gaudet is the Executive Director of Duke Integrative Medicine at Duke University Medical Center in Durham, North Carolina. Under her leadership, Duke Integrative Medicine has recently opened a state-of-the-art health care facility dedicated to the transformation of medicine through the exploration of new models of whole-person health care. Prior to her work at Duke, Dr. Gaudet was the founding Executive Director of the University of Arizona Program in Integrative Medicine, helping to design the country's first comprehensive curriculum in this new field. Dr. Gaudet is the author of *Consciously Female*, a book on integrative medicine and women's health, and *Body, Soul, and Baby*, a comprehensive guide to pregnancy. She writes a regular column for *Body+Soul* magazine and is widely recognized as a leader in the emerging field of integrative medicine through her contributions to numerous journals, publications, and television programs.

William W. George
Bill George is a Professor of Management Practice at Harvard Business School, where he is teaching leadership and leadership development, and

is the Henry B. Arthur Fellow of Ethics. He is the author of the best-selling books *True North, Discover Your Authentic Leadership* and *Authentic Leadership: Rediscovering the Secrets of Creating Lasting Value.* Mr. George is the former Chairman and CEO of Medtronic. Under his leadership, Medtronic's market capitalization grew from $1.1 billion to $60 billion, averaging a 35 percent increase each year. Mr. George has made frequent appearances on television and radio, and his articles have appeared in numerous publications. He has been named one of "Top 25 Business Leaders of the Past 25 Years" by PBS.

Elizabeth A. Goldblatt, Ph.D., M.P.A./H.A.
(planning committee member)
Dr. Goldblatt is Chair of the Academic Consortium for Complementary and Alternative Health Care. She is currently Vice President for Academic Affairs at the American College of Traditional Chinese Medicine (ACTCM), and she was President of the Council of Colleges of Acupuncture and Oriental Medicine from 1996 to 2002. She oversees an integrative clinical doctoral program at ACTCM, and works with the University of California Osher Center and California Pacific Medical Center in acupuncture internship placements and developing cross-education projects. Dr. Goldblatt believes that when the biomedical community and the complementary alternative medicine community build health care teams and work collaboratively in integrative settings, that this approach to health care is often best for the patient's treatment and healing process.

Lawrence W. Green, Dr.P.H.
Dr. Green, before joining the University of California, San Francisco, was Director of the Office of Science and Extramural Research for the Centers for Disease Control. He has been on the public health and medical faculties at University of California, Berkeley; Johns Hopkins University, Harvard University, University of Texas, Houston, and the University of British Columbia. He was the first Director of the Office of Health Promotion under the Carter administration, and a Vice President of the Henry J. Kaiser Family Foundation. He has published several books and over 300 articles on program planning, evidence, and evaluation issues in health services and public health. He has served on the U.S. Preventive Services Task Force and now serves on the Task Force on Community Preventive Services as Associate Editor of the *Annual Reviews of Public Health*, and on the editorial boards of 13 other journals.

Erminia "Mimi" Guarneri, M.D., FACC
(planning committee member)
Dr. Guarneri is the Founder and Medical Director of the Scripps Center for Integrative Medicine. Recognizing the need for a more comprehensive and more holistic approach to cardiovascular disease, she pioneered the center where she uses state-of-the-art cardiac imaging technology and lifestyle change programs to aggressively diagnose, prevent, and treat cardiovascular disease. She is the author of *The Heart Speaks*, a poignant collection of stories from heart patients who have benefited from integrative medicine approaches. Dr. Guarneri is regularly quoted in national publications such as the *Yoga Journal, Body+Soul* magazine and *WebMD*. Her medical degree is from SUNY Medical Center in New York where she graduated number one in her class.

George C. Halvorson
Mr. Halvorson was named Chairman and CEO of Kaiser Foundation Health Plan, Inc., and Kaiser Foundation Hospitals in March 2002. He was formerly President and CEO of HealthPartners, headquartered in Minneapolis. He is the author of comprehensive books on the U.S. health care system including his latest, *Health Care Reform Now!* In January 2009, Mr. Halvorson chaired the Healthcare Governor's Meeting of the World Economic Forum in Davos, Switzerland. He serves on a number of boards, including those of America's Health Insurance Plans, where he was the 2007 to 2008 Chair, and the Alliance of Community Health Plans. He is the current President of the International Federation of Health Plans and Chair of the Partnership for Quality Care with the Service Employees International Union. George also serves on the Institute of Medicine's Roundtable on Evidence-Based Medicine and on the Commonwealth Fund's Commission on a High-Performance Health System. Widely credited with supporting the successful rollout of Kaiser's multibillion dollar information technology initiative, Mr. Halvorson has won numerous awards for his commitment to health technology, including the Modern Healthcare CEO IT Achievement Award.

Senator Tom Harkin
Since first being elected to the U.S. Congress in 1974 and later to the U.S. Senate in 1984, Senator Tom Harkin (D-IA) has led the fight to improve health care for every American, including those in rural areas and people with disabilities. Concerned by reports of rising obesity and pre-

ventable illness, Harkin has introduced the Healthy Lifestyles and Prevention America Act, which takes a comprehensive approach encouraging healthier lifestyles and focusing on nutrition, physical activity, mental health, and tobacco cessation. Recently, Senator Edward Kennedy tapped Harkin to lead a working group charged with crafting the prevention and public health components of the upcoming health reform bill. Harkin is currently the Chairman of the Senate Labor, Health and Human Services, and Education Appropriations Subcommittee, the Chairman of the Senate Agriculture, Nutrition and Forestry Committee, as well as being a senior member on the Senate Health, Education, Labor and Pension Committee and the Small Business Committee.

Michael M. E. Johns, M.D.
(planning committee member)
Dr. Johns assumed the post of Chancellor for Emory University on October 1, 2007. Prior to that, starting in 1996, he served as Executive Vice President for Health Affairs; CEO, the Robert W. Woodruff Health Sciences Center; Chairman of the Board, Emory Healthcare; Cochairman of the Board, EHCA, LLC; and Professor, Department of Otolaryngology, Emory University School of Medicine. Dr. Johns engineered the transformation of the Health Sciences Center into one of the nation's preeminent centers in education, research, and patient care. Highlights include major growth and reshaping of the research enterprise, development of enhanced curricula for each of the health professions schools, formation of Emory Healthcare through consolidation and realignment of Emory's extensive clinical enterprise, and the most extensive facilities improvement plan in Emory history. Dr. Johns received his bachelor's degree at Wayne State University and his medical degree from the University of Michigan Medical School. As a cancer surgeon of head and neck tumors, he was internationally recognized for his clinical care and his studies of treatment outcomes.

Janet R. Kahn, Ph.D.
Dr. Kahn is Executive Director of the Integrated Healthcare Policy Consortium (www.ihpc.info), Director of the Center for Integrated Health Care at the Community Health Center of Burlington, and Research Assistant Professor in the Department of Psychiatry at the University of Vermont. She is a medical sociologist with an interest in the organizational issues of equitable health care delivery and the role of federal, state, and local policies on individual health-related choices. She is also a

massage therapist, specializing in treating people with chronic pain and exploring the contributions of touch, movement, and mindfulness to human well-being. Dr. Kahn is a coinvestigator on two studies currently in the field—a clinical trial comparing forms of massage with different theoretical mechanisms of action for treatment of chronic low back pain, and a Phase II Small Business Innovation Research grant to develop and test an educational DVD and print manual for cancer patients and their caregivers.

David L. Katz, M.D., M.P.H., FACPM, FACP

Dr. Katz is an internationally recognized authority on nutrition, weight management, and the prevention of chronic disease. He is a board certified specialist in both Internal Medicine and Preventive Medicine/Public Health, and Associate Professor (adjunct) in Public Health Practice at the Yale University School of Medicine. Katz is the Director and Founder of Yale University's Prevention Research Center and the Integrative Medicine Center at Griffin Hospital in Derby, Connecticut, as well as Founder and President of the nonprofit Turn the Tide Foundation. Katz has published over 100 scientific papers and chapters and 12 books to date; he has acquired and managed some $25 million in research funds. He is a prominent medical journalist and commentator, having formerly served as a medical contributor to ABC News with routine appearances on *Good Morning America*. The owner of five U.S. patents, Katz is the principal inventor of the Overall Nutritional Quality Index (ONQI) algorithm (www.nuval.com).

Mary Jo Kreitzer, Ph.D., R.N., FAAN

Dr. Kreitzer is Founder and Director of the Center for Spirituality and Healing. She is currently the coprincipal investigator of several clinical trials and grants that encompass a variety of topics: mindfulness meditation for solid organ transplant patients; integrated residential treatment programs for women with eating disorders; mind–body interventions for caregivers of Alzheimer's patients; comparing mindfulness meditation with pharmacotherapy for people with chronic insomnia; and integrating research in a complementary and alternative medicine educational institution. In addition to her administrative responsibilities in the Center for Spirituality and Healing, Dr. Kreitzer teaches in the graduate minor in complementary therapies and healing practices and is a tenured professor in the School of Nursing. From 2004 to 2007, she served as the Vice Chair of the Consortium of Academic Health Centers for Integrative

Medicine. She was recently named by Minnesota Physician as one of the 100 most influential health care leaders in the state. Dr. Kreitzer earned her doctoral degree in health services research and her master's and bachelor's degrees in nursing.

Richard Lifton, M.D., Ph.D.
(planning committee member)
Richard Lifton is Chairman of the Department of Genetics, Sterling Professor of Genetics and Internal Medicine, Director of the Yale Center for Human Genetics and Genomics, and Investigator of the Howard Hughes Medical Institute at Yale University School of Medicine. Dr. Lifton's laboratory has used human genetics and genomics to identify causes of heart, kidney, and bone disease. By investigating thousands of families from around the world, his group has identified more than 25 human disease genes. These include key genes and pathways that are critical to the risk of hypertension, stroke, heart attack, and osteoporosis. These studies have provided new diagnostic and therapeutic approaches to these diseases, which affect more than 1 billion people worldwide. His honors include election to the National Academy of Sciences, the Institute of Medicine, and the 2008 Wiley Prize in Biomedical Sciences.

Mike Magee, M.D.
Dr. Magee is Senior Fellow for Health Policy at the Center for Aging Services Technologies of the American Association of Homes and Services for the Aging and Editor of HealthCommentary.org and Healthy-Waters.org. He is well known for his unique perspective on health care and for the championing of patient rights, principled leadership, access to scientific discoveries, and a populist vision for health system reform in the United States. From 2003 to 2007, Dr. Magee was the host of *Health Politics with Dr. Mike Magee*, a weekly Internet program covering news and information related to health and health care, which covered a range of topics from obesity to aging and caregiving to global warming. He is the author of 10 books, including *Home-Centered Health Care, Positive Leadership,* and *Healthy Waters*. Dr. Magee is a member of the National Commission for Quality Long-Term Care, chaired by former U.S. Senator Bob Kerrey and former U.S. House Speaker Newt Gingrich.

Victoria Maizes, M.D.
Dr. Maizes is Executive Director of the Arizona Center for Integrative Medicine at the University of Arizona and an Associate Professor of

Medicine, Family, and Community Medicine and Public Health. As founding Cochair of the education committee of the Consortium of Academic Health Centers for Integrative Medicine, Dr. Maizes led a team of educators developing objectives for medical students in integrative medicine. Dr. Maizes stewarded the growth of the Program in Integrative Medicine from a small program educating four residential fellows per year to a designated Center of Excellence training more than 150 residents and fellows in its comprehensive integrative medicine educational programs. She helped create the comprehensive curriculum in integrative medicine that is now used for fellows and pioneered multiple innovative educational programs including the Integrative Family Medicine Program and Integrative Medicine in Residency, two national models for educating primary care physicians. She is frequently sought out as a speaker on topics including integrative medical education, women's health, healthy aging, nutrition, and cancer.

Bruce S. McEwen, Ph.D.
(planning committee member)
Dr. McEwen is the Alfred E. Mirsky Professor and Head of the Harold and Margaret Milliken Hatch Laboratory of Neuroendocrinology at the Rockefeller University. As a neuroscientist and neuroendocrinologist, McEwen studies environmentally regulated, variable gene expression in the brain mediated by circulating steroid hormones and endogenous neurotransmitters in relation to brain sexual differentiation and the actions of sex, stress, and thyroid hormones on the adult brain. His laboratory discovered adrenal steroid receptors in the hippocampus in 1968. His laboratory combines molecular, anatomical, pharmacological, physiological, and behavioral methodologies and relates their findings to human clinical information. His current research focuses on stress effects on amygdala and prefrontal cortex as well as hippocampus, and his laboratory also investigates sex hormone effects and sex differences in these brain regions.

Arnold Milstein M.D., M.P.H.
Dr. Milstein is the Medical Director of the Pacific Business Group on Health and the Chief Physician at Mercer Health & Benefits. His work and publications focus on health care purchasing strategy, the psychology of clinical performance improvement, and clinical innovations that reduce total health care spending. He cofounded both the Leapfrog Group and the Consumer-Purchaser Disclosure Project. He heads

performance measurement activities for both initiatives and is a Congressional MedPAC Commissioner. The *New England Journal of Medicine*'s series on employer-sponsored health insurance described him as a "pioneer" in efforts to advance quality of care. He was selected for the highest annual award of the National Business Group on Health, for nationally distinguished innovation in health care cost reduction and quality gains.

William Novelli
Mr. Novelli is CEO of AARP, a membership organization of 40 million people age 50 and older, half of whom remain actively employed. Prior to joining AARP, Mr. Novelli was President of the Campaign for Tobacco-Free Kids. Previously, he was Executive Vice President of CARE, the world's largest private relief and development organization. Earlier, Mr. Novelli cofounded and was President of Porter Novelli, now one of the world's largest public relations agencies and part of the Omnicom Group, an international marketing communications corporation. He retired from the firm in 1990 to pursue a second career in public service. He was named one of the 100 most influential public relations professionals of the 20th century by the industry's leading publication. Mr. Novelli is a recognized leader in social marketing and social change, and has managed programs in cancer control, diet and nutrition, cardiovascular health, reproductive health, infant survival, pay increases for educators, charitable giving, and other programs in the United States and the developing world.

Dean Ornish, M.D.
(planning committee member)
Dr. Ornish is the Founder and President of the nonprofit Preventive Medicine Research Institute (www.pmri.org), where he holds the Safeway Chair, and he is Clinical Professor of Medicine at the University of California, San Francisco. For over 30 years, Dr. Ornish has directed randomized controlled trials demonstrating, for the first time, that comprehensive lifestyle changes may begin to reverse even severe coronary heart disease and early-stage prostate cancer without drugs or surgery. He and his colleagues recently demonstrated that comprehensive lifestyle changes may up-regulate disease-preventing genes and down-regulate genes that promote cancer and heart disease. This study also showed, for the first time, that comprehensive lifestyle changes may increase telomerase and, thus, telomeres, the ends of chromosomes that

control how long we live. He is the author of six best-selling books, including his newest *New York Times'* bestseller, *The Spectrum*. Dr. Ornish was selected as one of the *"TIME* 100" in integrative medicine and chosen by *LIFE* magazine as "one of the fifty most influential members of his generation."

Mehmet C. Oz, M.D.

Dr. Oz is the Vice Chair and Professor of Surgery at Columbia University. His research interests include heart replacement surgery, minimally invasive cardiac surgery, complementary medicine, and health care policy. He has authored over 400 original publications, book chapters, and medical books, and he has received several patents. He performs an estimated 250 heart operations annually. Dr. Oz is the Health Expert on *The Oprah Winfrey Show* and is also host of *The Doctor Oz Show* heard daily on *Oprah & Friends*—SiriusXM Radio. He has been the chief medical consultant to Discovery Communications, and his *Transplant!* series won both a Freddie and a Silver Telly award. In addition to numerous appearances on *Good Morning America*, he has guest hosted *The Charlie Rose Show* and appeared on all the evening news broadcasts. In addition to belonging to every major professional society for heart surgeons, Dr. Oz has been honored as one of *Time* magazine's 100 Most Influential People (2008) and *Esquire* magazine's 75 Most Influential People of the 21st century.

Kenneth R. Pelletier, Ph.D., M.D.(hc)

Dr. Pelletier is a Clinical Professor of Medicine and Professor of Public Health at the University of Arizona School of Medicine and Director of the Corporate Health Improvement Program (CHIP). He is also a Clinical Professor of Medicine in the Departments of Family and Community Medicine and Psychiatry at the University of California School of Medicine (UCSF) San Francisco. Prior to these positions, Dr. Pelletier served as Clinical Professor of Medicine, Stanford University School of Medicine; Director of the Stanford Corporate Health Program; and was Director of the NIH-funded Complementary and Alternative Medicine Program at Stanford (CAMPS). He was a Woodrow Wilson Fellow, studied at the C.G. Jung Institute in Zurich, Switzerland, and has published over 300 professional journal articles in behavioral medicine, disease management, worksite interventions, and alternative/integrative medicine. At the present time, Dr. Pelletier is a medical and business advisor to the World Health Organization (WHO), the National Business Group on

Health, the Federation of State Medical Boards, and several national and international corporations including Ford, Dow, IBM, Prudential, Pepsi, and NASA. Dr. Pelletier is the author of 12 major books including the international bestseller *New Medicine: Integrating Complementary, Alternative, and Conventional Medicine.*

Adam Perlman, M.D., M.P.H., FACP

Dr. Perlman became Director of Integrative Medicine for the Saint Barnabas Health Care System and founding Medical Director for the Carol and Morton Siegler Center for Integrative Medicine, in Livingston, New Jersey, in 1998. In that role, he had primary responsibility for developing and overseeing the Complementary and Alternative Medicine Program for the largest health care system in New Jersey. In 2002, Dr. Perlman became Executive Director for the Institute for Complementary and Alternative Medicine (ICAM) at the University of Medicine and Dentistry of New Jersey (UMDNJ), where he is an Associate Professor of Medicine. In 2004, he was named the UMDNJ Hunterdon Endowed Professor in Complementary and Alternative Medicine; and in 2007, Dr. Perlman was appointed Chairperson for the Department of Primary Care within the School of Health-Related Professions. In that role, he oversees the Physician Assistant Program and Respiratory Care Program in addition to the Institute for Complementary and Alternative Medicine.

Victor S. Sierpina, M.D.
(planning committee member)
Dr. Sierpina is Professor of Family Medicine with tenure at the University of Texas Medical Branch (UTMB) in Galveston, Texas. He is the first designated W.D. and Laura Nell Nicholson Family Professor of Integrative Medicine at UTMB. He graduated from the University of Illinois Abraham Lincoln School of Medicine as a James Scholar and completed family practice residency at MacNeal Memorial Hospital in suburban Chicago. Since medical school, he has integrated holistic medicine, alternative therapies, and wellness promotion in primary care. Dr. Sierpina is board certified by the American Board of Family Medicine and the American Board of Holistic Medicine. He was recently recognized as one of the Best Doctors in the USA in *Family Medicine.* He is recipient of two NIH grants supporting his educational and research efforts in integrative medicine.

Ralph Snyderman, M.D.
(planning committee chair)
Dr. Snyderman is Chancellor Emeritus, Duke University and James B. Duke Professor of Medicine in the Duke University School of Medicine. He served as Chancellor for Health Affairs and Dean of the School of Medicine from 1989 to July 2004. Dr. Snyderman oversaw the development of the Duke University Health System, one of the most successful integrated academic health systems in the country, and served as its first President and CEO. Dr. Snyderman has been widely recognized for his contributions to the development of more rational, effective, and compassionate models of health care. He was awarded the first Bravewell Leadership Award for outstanding achievements in the field of integrative medicine in 2003. Snyderman has played a prominent role in the leadership of such important national organizations as the Association of American Physicians, the Institute of Medicine (IOM) and the Association of American Medical Colleges. He is a member of the IOM and the American Academy of Arts & Sciences.

Esther M. Sternberg, M.D.
(planning committee member)
Dr. Sternberg is internationally recognized for her discoveries in brain-immune interactions and the effects of the brain's stress response on health: the science of the mind–body interaction. Dr. Sternberg received her M.D. degree and trained in rheumatology at McGill University and was on the faculty at Washington University before joining the National Institutes of Health in 1986, where she is currently based. Her numerous original scientific and review articles and textbook chapters are published in leading scientific journals including *Science, Nature Reviews Immunology, Nature Medicine,* the *New England Journal of Medicine, Scientific American,* and *Proceedings of the National Academy of Sciences.* In addition, she is reviewer and editorial board member for many scientific journals, has edited several books, and authored the popular book *The Balance Within: The Science Connecting Health and Emotions.* Dr. Sternberg lectures nationally and internationally to both lay and scientific audiences and is frequently interviewed on radio, television, and film and in print media on subjects including the mind–body connection, stress and illness, and spirituality, love, and health. Her work galvanized establishment of the field of brain-immune interactions. In recognition of her accomplishments, Dr. Sternberg is one of 300 women physicians featured in the National Library of Medicine exhibition on women in medi-

cine: "Changing the Face of Medicine" (www.nlm.nih.gov/changingthe faceofmedicine/, click "Explore the Exhibition").

Ellen L. Stovall
(planning committee member)
Ms. Stovall is a 37-year survivor of three bouts with cancer. In 1992, she became President and CEO of the National Coalition for Cancer Survivorship (NCCS), a survivor-led organization that advocates for quality cancer care for all Americans and empowers people with cancer to advocate for themselves. Ms. Stovall is on the Board of the National Committee for Quality Assurance and has participated in working groups and committees advising the National Cancer Institute, American Association for Cancer Research, American Board of Internal Medicine, American Society of Clinical Oncology, and many other national organizations concerned with providing quality health care. She also served for six years as a presidential appointee to the National Cancer Advisory Board (NCAB). As a Vice Chair of the Institute of Medicine's National Cancer Policy Forum survivorship committee, Ms. Stovall co-edited the November 2005 report, *From Cancer Patient to Cancer Survivor: Lost in Transition*, which recommends comprehensive, coordinated follow-up care for people surviving a cancer diagnosis.

Kenneth E. Thorpe, Ph.D.
Dr. Thorpe is the Robert W. Woodruff Professor and Chair of the Department of Health Policy & Management in the Rollins School of Public Health of Emory University. He also codirects the Emory Center on Health Outcomes and Quality. He was previously Professor of Health Policy and Administration at the University of North Carolina at Chapel Hill, an Associate Professor and Director of the Program on Health Care Financing and Insurance at the Harvard University School of Public Health, and Assistant Professor of Public Policy and Public Health at Columbia University. Professor Thorpe was Deputy Assistant Secretary for Health Policy in the U.S. Department of Health and Human Services from 1993 to 1995. In this capacity, he coordinated all financial estimates and program impacts of President Clinton's health care reform proposals for the White House. He also directed the administration's estimation efforts in dealing with Congressional health care reform proposals during the 103rd and 104th sessions of Congress.

Reed V. Tuckson, M.D., FACP
(planning committee member)
Dr. Tuckson is currently Executive Vice President and Chief of Medical Affairs at UnitedHealth Group. He is responsible for working with all of the company's business units to improve the quality and efficiency of health services. Formerly, Dr. Tuckson served as Senior Vice President, Professional Standards, for the American Medical Association. He is former President of the Charles R. Drew University of Medicine and Science in Los Angeles; has served as Senior Vice President for Programs of the March of Dimes Birth Defects Foundation; and is a former Commissioner of Public Health for the District of Columbia. Dr. Tuckson was featured on the cover of the February 2009 issue of *Black Enterprise* magazine and named one of the 100 Most Powerful Executives in Corporate America. Last year, he was named one of *Modern Healthcare*'s Top 25 Minority Executives in Healthcare for 2008 and to *Ebony* magazine's 2008 Power 150: The Most Influential Blacks in America list.

Sean Tunis, M.D., M.Sc.
(planning committee member)
Dr. Tunis is the Founder and Director of the Center for Medical Technology Policy. Through September of 2005, Dr. Tunis was the Director of the Office of Clinical Standards and Quality and Chief Medical Officer at the Centers for Medicare and Medicaid Services (CMS). Dr. Tunis served as the Senior Advisor to the CMS Administrator on clinical and scientific policy, and he supervised the development of national coverage policies; quality standards for Medicare and Medicaid providers; quality measurement and public reporting initiatives; and the Quality Improvement Organization program. Before joining CMS, Dr. Tunis was a Senior Research Scientist with the Lewin Group, where his focus was on the design and implementation of prospective comparative effectiveness trials and clinical registries. Dr. Tunis also served as the Director of the Health Program at the Congressional Office of Technology Assessment and as a Health Policy Advisor to the U.S. Senate Committee on Labor and Human Resources, where he participated in policy development regarding pharmaceutical and device regulation.

Edward H. Wagner, M.D., M.P.H., FACP
Dr. Wagner is a general internist/epidemiologist and Director of the MacColl Institute for Healthcare Innovation at Group Health Center for Health Studies. His research and quality improvement work focus on

improving the care of seniors and others with chronic illness. Since 1998, he has directed Improving Chronic Illness Care, a national program of the Robert Wood Johnson Foundation. He and his MacColl Institute colleagues developed the Chronic Care Model, which now serves as the foundation for improving ambulatory care for many organizations nationally and internationally. He also is Principal Investigator of the Cancer Research Network, a National Cancer Institute-funded cancer research consortium of 14 HMO-based research programs. He has written two books and more than 250 published articles.

STAFF BIOGRAPHIES

Katharine Bothner

Ms. Bothner is a research associate in the Institute of Medicine's Exccutive Office, where she has worked on a number of projects, including *HHS in the 21st Century: Charting a New Course for a Healthier America*, the Summit on Integrative Medicine and the Health of the Public, and the Robert Wood Johnson Foundation Initiative on the Future of Nursing, at the IOM. She began working with the IOM in October 2006 as a senior program assistant with the Roundtable on Evidence-Based Medicine. She received a B.S. in chemistry with high distinction from the University of Virginia in 2004 and conducted her thesis research on a cytostatic cancer therapy involving calcium channels. After completing her undergraduate studies, Ms. Bothner taught high school science for 2 years in Baltimore, Maryland, with Teach for America. More than 70 percent of her 10th-grade biology students passed the Maryland High School Assessment test, a figure nearly twice the city average.

Samantha M. Chao, M.P.H.

Ms. Chao is a Program Officer at the Institute of Medicine. Her work focuses on improving health care quality with a focus on patient-centered care. She has directed the IOM's Forum on the Science of Health Care Quality Improvement and Implementation and worked on the IOM's *Pathways to Quality Health Care* project. The forum convened stakeholders from the government, academia, and industry to improve the quality and value of health care through the strengthening of quality improvement and implementation research. The *Pathways* series consisted of a review of performance measures to analyze health care delivery, an evaluation of Medicare's Quality Improvement Organization Program, and an assessment of pay-for-performance and its potential role in Medicare. Prior to joining the IOM, she completed a master's degree in health policy with a concentration in management at the University of Michigan School of Public Health. As part of her studies, she interned with the American Heart Association, where she helped develop the association's position on pay-for-performance. She also worked with the Michigan Department of Community Health to promote the study of chronic disease and disease prevention.

J. Michael McGinnis, M.D., M.P.P.

Dr. McGinnis is a physician and long-time contributor to national and international health policy leadership. Since 2005 he has been Senior Scholar at the Institute of Medicine (IOM), leading its initiative on evidence and value-based health care. He is also an elected member of the IOM. From 1999 to 2005, Dr. McGinnis was Senior Vice President and founding health group director at the Robert Wood Johnson Foundation. Previously, and, unusual for political posts, he held continuous appointment through the Carter, Reagan, Bush, and Clinton administrations at the U.S. Department of Health and Human Services, with policy responsibilities for disease prevention and health promotion (1977–1995). His international work includes service in 1995–1996 as Chair of the World Bank/European Commission Health Reconstruction Task Force in Bosnia, and in 1974–1975 as epidemiologist and state director for World Health Organization's smallpox eradication program in India.

Judith A. Salerno, M.D., M.S.

Dr. Salerno is executive officer of the Institute of Medicine of the National Academies. Dr. Salerno served as deputy director of the National Institute on Aging (NIA) at the National Institutes of Health from 2001 to 2007, where she had oversight of more than $1 billion in aging research conducted and supported annually by the NIA, including research on Alzheimer's and other neurodegenerative diseases; frailty and function in late life; and the social, behavioral, and demographic aspects of aging. A geriatrician, Dr. Salerno is vitally interested in improving the health and well-being of older persons, and has designed public-private initiatives to address aging stereotypes, novel approaches to support training of new investigators in aging, and award-winning programs to communicate health and research advances to the public. Before joining the NIA in 2001, Dr. Salerno directed the continuum of geriatrics and extended care programs across the country for the U.S. Department of

Veterans Affairs (VA), Washington, D.C. While at the VA, she launched widely recognized national initiatives for pain management and improving end-of-life care and directed a national program of geriatric and long-term care services of more than $3 billion annually. Dr. Salerno earned her M.D. degree from Harvard Medical School in 1985 and a master of science degree in health policy from the Harvard School of Public Health in 1976. She also holds a certificate of added qualifications in geriatric medicine and was associate clinical professor of health care sciences and of medicine at the George Washington University until 2001.

Andrea M. Schultz, M.P.H.
Ms. Schultz is an associate program officer in the Executive Office of the Institute of Medicine. Ms. Schultz joined the Board on Health Sciences Policy in 2004 where she worked on a number of reports, including *Genes, Behavior, and the Social Environment: Moving Beyond the Nature/Nurture Debate*; *Reusability of Facemasks During an Influenza Pandemic: Facing the Flu*; *Organ Donation: Opportunities for Action*; and *Cord Blood: Establishing a National Hematopoietic Stem Cell Bank Program*. In 2006 she moved to the IOM's Executive Office and Office of Reports and Communications where she provided health policy research support on a variety of issues for the IOM president and executive officer, coordinated an effort to collect and catalog impact data on IOM reports, and helped lead the IOM's Quality Improvement effort. Under the Executive Office, Ms. Schultz recently worked on *HHS in the 21st Century: Charting a New Course for a Healthier America*, and she is currently working on the Summit on Integrative Medicine and the Health of the Public and the Robert Wood Johnson Foundation Initiative on the Future of Nursing at the Institute of Medicine. She received her M.P.H. in health policy with honors in August 2007 from George Washington University. Her capstone project analyzed key state-level health care reform initiatives. Ms. Schultz received her B.S. in cellular molecular biology from the University of Michigan in 2004.

Joi D. Washington
Ms. Washington is a Senior Program Assistant for the Board on Health Care Services. Prior to joining the IOM in May 2008, Ms. Washington held the position of Registrar at the National Minority AIDS Council in which she oversaw the registration process for two large national conferences. Ms. Washington received her B.S. in Public and Community Health from the University of Maryland, College Park, in 2007

and is currently pursuing a dual master's degree in Health Care Administration and Business Administration from the University of Maryland, University College.

Catherine Zweig

Ms. Zweig is a Senior Program Assistant for the Roundtable on Evidence Based Medicine. She received a B.A. in Government from Colby College (Magna Cum Laude) where she also had a concentration in Chemistry. Ms. Zweig focused on foreign development in college and wrote her honors thesis on public opinion polling as a tool for building peace in the Niger Delta region of Nigeria. She also cochaired the Student Advisory Board at the Goldfarb Center for Public Affairs and Civic Engagement, Colby's primary focus for outreach and leader involvement. Ms. Zweig joined the staff of the Institute of Medicine's Roundtable on Evidence-Based Medicine in the summer of 2008.

E

Issue Background Material

The Institute of Medicine commissioned several papers as background material for the Summit on Integrative Medicine and the Health of the Public (see Box E-1 below). Those papers can be accessed on the summit's website: www.iom.edu/integrativemedicine. Reflective of the varied range of issues and interpretations related to integrative medicine, the papers developed represent a broad range of perspectives. Summarized below, by consultant Vicki Weisfeld, are key elements on those topics.

As with each commissioned activity, the responsibility for the content rests solely with the authors and does not necessarily represent the views or endorsement of the Institute of Medicine or its committees and convening bodies.

BOX E-1
Commissioned Background Material for the Summit

IOM Summit on Integrative Medicine and the Health of the Public: Issue Background and Overview
Vicki Weisfeld

Integrative Medicine Research: Context and Priorities
Gary Deng, M.D., Ph.D.
Wendy Weber, N.D., Ph.D., M.P.H.
Amit Sood, M.D., M.Sc.
Kathi Kemper, M.D., M.P.H.

Preventive Medicine, Integrative Medicine, and the Health of the Public
David L. Katz, M.D., M.P.H., FACPM, FACP
Ather Ali, N.D., M.P.H.

Integrative Medicine and Patient-Centered Care
Victoria Maizes, M.D.
David Rakel, M.D.
Catherine Niemiec, J.D., L.Ac.

Health Professions Education and Integrative Health Care
Mary Jo Kreitzer, Ph.D., R.N., FAAN
Benjamin Kligler, M.D., M.P.H.
William C. Meeker, D.C., M.P.H.

Communicating with the Public about Integrative Medicine
Susan Bauer-Wu, Ph.D., R.N.
Mary Ruggie, Ph.D.
Matt Russell

Health and Medical Economics: Applications to Integrative Medicine
Kenneth R. Pelletier, Ph.D., M.D. (hc)
Patricia M. Herman, N.D., Ph.D.
R. Douglas Metz, D.C.
Craig F. Nelson, D.C.

PATIENT-CENTERED CARE

Patient-centered care is one of the six aims for a 21st-century health care system recommended in the IOM report, *Crossing the Quality Chasm* care "respectful of and responsive to individual patient preferences, needs, and values and ensuring that patient values guide all clinical decisions" (IOM, 2001). A health system that achieved patient-centered care and the report's other five aims (care that is safe, effective, timely, efficient, and equitable) would, the authors write, enable patients to count on receiving the full array of preventive, acute, and chronic services likely to benefit them. The following several specific "rules" identified for a redesigned health system would increase patient-centeredness and parallel the goals of integrative medicine:

- Customization of care based on patient needs and values
- Giving patients the necessary information and the opportunity for shared decision making

- Shared knowledge and information between patients and clinicians
- Transparency of information for patients choosing health plans, hospitals, clinical practices, or alternative treatments
- Anticipating patient needs—a concept that should include disease prevention and health promotion—rather than simply reacting to events

Each of these is important to the vision of integrative medicine, which expands the notion of patient-centeredness to a coordinated approach to delivery along with a careful consideration of the family, social, and community dynamics that can shape the course of the healing processes. Achieving a system responsive to patients in this way would require qualitatively different communication between patients and their health care providers, as well as giving patients a more central role in managing their own health prospects and disease treatment.

Programs encouraging self-management of such chronic conditions as diabetes or asthma are examples of trends that mirror the concepts of integrative medicine. These programs have developed some best-practice approaches for engaging patients, encouraging greater patient responsibility for health maintenance, encouraging their greater role, and drawing on supportive community programs. They include individual consultation with physicians who provide state-of-the-art treatment; health education and nutrition counseling by nurses, nutritionists, and others; and individual and group counseling and support. Such comprehensive approaches have been shown to improve health outcomes, reduce hospitalizations and emergency room visits, and save costs. Such comprehensive models as these may be replicable for other chronic conditions.

The medical home concept currently is being advanced by four specialty societies for primary care physicians, which have issued joint principles intended to operationalize the patient-centered medical home.[1] Many integrative medicine concepts are embraced by this approach. The principles advocate that

- each patient should have an ongoing relationship with a physician trained to provide comprehensive care;

---

[1] American Academy of Family Physicians, American Academy of Pediatrics, American College of Physicians, and American Osteopathic Association, together representing approximately 333,000 physicians.

- this physician should lead a team that collectively takes ongoing responsibility for the patient's care;
- the physician should have a whole-person, whole-life orientation;
- care should be coordinated and integrated across all elements of the health care system;
- care provided should be high quality and safe;
- patients should have greater electronic and other access to their practice; and
- the payment system should reward the added value that having a medical home offers patients.

A patient-centered approach relies on the notion of multidisciplinary teams working in a seamless integrated fashion. Team members provide appropriate components of care and counseling that fit their skills and training and reasonably limit costly physician time. Certain team members can be responsible for regular patient monitoring, mentoring and educational reinforcement, and psychosocial support, which enhance continuity of care. Teams also may include patient navigators to help patients access different health system components. Similarly, some model medical home projects that provide comprehensive services hire LPNs with deep community knowledge and good communications skills to conduct home visits and patient education. Through them, the medical practice learns a great deal about the patient's home environment and what is practical and possible in the way of self-management and lifestyle change.

A major factor impeding the diffusion of patient-centered, integrated care models is the current reimbursement system, which undervalues primary care and preventive counscling services and overvalues procedure-intensive specialty care. The number of medical students choosing primary care has dropped precipitously, and this financial discrepancy is cited by many as a principal reason for pursuing specialty training. This trend runs directly counter to ample evidence from the United States and abroad that communities with high proportions of primary care providers have better health, including lower death rates, than communities whose physician complement is dominated by specialists. Hospitals and academic medical centers have little incentive to promote primary care, because it does not bring in the high reimbursements and research dollars that specialty care does, and subsidies for primary care residency training are lower.

The procedure-oriented health system is geared toward disease events, rather than patient-centered care, and change is hard. Health care providers have a legacy of paternalistic attitudes toward patients that, in turn, have fostered a generation or more of passive patients. Large numbers of Americans are not health literate, let alone health proficient. The growing number of immigrants including many people who are not proficient in English increases the challenge. Effectively involving culturally diverse groups with the health care system, before of after the onset of disease, is difficult.

Provider culture is also a challenge to patient-centered care. Despite years of discussing the importance of teamwork in providing effective health care services, health professions training and the professionalization process (and, sometimes, state scope-of-practice laws) inhibit the development of flexible, mutually supportive team-based care. Again, *Crossing the Quality Chasm* notes that, although team-based care is common at least in theory, its full benefits are inhibited by traditional roles, and it is "slowed or stymied by institutional, labor, and financial structures, and by law and custom" (IOM, 2001).

Greater appreciation of these challenges offers prospects for change. Health reform efforts will likely seek to shift economic incentives toward primary care and prevention. Wider use of health information technology is expected to increase the efficiency, effectiveness, continuity, and integration of the care process. Electronic health records (EHR), which are gradually increasing in U.S. health care and promoted in the February 2009 economic stimulus legislation, will offer an important tool to facilitate providers' and patients' ability to obtain the information needed to the right place at the right time, with electronic prompts and decision aids. Moreover, greater access by patients to Web-based information on diagnostic and treatment protocols will deepen the capacity and motivation for patients to seek tailored information about their health condition—information that may help center patient and provider discussions around key issues.

PREVENTION AND HEALTH OF THE PUBLIC

Preventive medicine and public health share the objectives of promoting general health, preventing diseases, and applying the techniques of epidemiology to achieving these ends. Preventive medicine focuses on individual patients, while public health uses organized community efforts to promote health in populations by, for example, increasing availability of healthful food choices or discouraging cigarette smoking.

Good health results from the complex interplay of genetic, behavioral, environmental, psychosocial, and health care factors. Health care services, per se, play a relatively small role as a determinant of a population's health. Even so, it is greatly beneficial for physicians to assess, encourage, and support modification of these factors, to the extent possible. With the increased capability of genomic medicine, physicians increasingly will be able to tailor educational and intervention efforts to the biological vulnerabilities and strengths of specific individuals.

Individual behavior—smoking, alcohol and drug abuse, lack of exercise, poor diet, reactions to stress, and so on—are the chief causes of poor health among Americans. More than 15 years ago, epidemiologic analysis yielded estimates that, in the United States, fully half of the mortality from the 10 leading causes of death was attributable to behavior that causes chronic diseases or makes them more serious (McGinnis and Foege, 1993). Lifestyle choices are a major contributor to development of heart disease, stroke, diabetes, some cancers, and injuries, including fires, falls, automobile injuries, suicide, and homicide. However, these choices are not made in a vacuum; a variety of social influences affect personal behavior. Modern preventive approaches have moved from a sole focus on persuading individuals to change their habits to altering the environment in ways that discourage negative behavior and encourage healthier decisions.

Clearly, the consequences of unhealthy behavior are costly, not only to individuals and families, but also for the entire health system. Disease prevention and wellness efforts cannot prevent every case of these diseases and injuries, but, even when disease occurs, they usually can help slow disease progress and avoid many serious sequelae. For example, a robust prevention-oriented approach to managing patients with diabetes can prevent foot and leg amputations and blindness.

Social and environmental influences on health come in many forms. Social factors include race, ethnicity, and minority or immigrant status. They also include family structure, income, education, and health insurance status. These factors clearly influence the development of young children, but they also affect levels of psychosocial stress and physical and mental health throughout life. Social factors, of course, also can be great sources of strength, and their positive potential can be marshaled to promote health. With respect to health insurance status, physicians rarely know anything about their patients' coverage and, therefore, the out-of-pocket cost burden specific recommendations may entail—perhaps one reason their advice is so frequently not followed.

Harmful environmental influences are factors in the physical environment, like exposures to harmful chemical or biological substances in air, water, food, or consumer products; excessive noise or sunlight (ultraviolet); or radiation from medical or occupational exposures. They include safety hazards to which people are exposed in the home, at work, and when traveling, especially in automobiles. Control of these factors lies more in the realm of public health practice and environmental design than in clinical medicine; however, a physician's awareness of the environment in which patients live and work can guide advice on risk mitigation. Such advice is particularly important for patients with genetic or other physical factors that might make environmental exposures more hazardous.

Since integrative medicine begins from the perspective of maintaining and promoting individual health, it is necessarily closely attuned to the array of behavioral and environmental factors that put health at risk. Inevitably, the health system must look beyond the individual patient to broader social and environmental influences. As mentioned, many environmental factors require public health advocacy and intervention. However, even individual behavior, such as smoking and exercise, is susceptible to social and environmental approaches. Widespread anti-smoking advocacy and supportive public policies, like anti-smoking rules in workplaces and public spaces, increased tobacco taxes, and consumer education programs have changed the environment in the United States from a pro-smoking to largely anti-smoking culture. Similarly, public policies that promote exercise by building bike, jogging, and walking trails; corporations and city planners that encourage office and residential buildings to include gyms and showers; and an array of other public policies support a health-promotion culture. Health professionals have credibility in public discussions of such policies and can do a great deal for their own patients and the community by endorsing such pro-health initiatives. Medical researchers and health policy analysts can develop the clinical research and public policy assessments on which sound public policies can be based.

HEALTH PROFESSIONS EDUCATION

The dominant emphasis on diagnosis and treatment of disease events by an increasingly specialized clinician workforce characterizes health care today. The integrative notions of tending to the whole patient, emphasizing wellness, engaging patients centrally in their care, and the related goals of fostering continuity of care and community health are clearly not the foci of most health professions education. Indeed, prevention and the holistic approach at the core of integrative medicine are substantially marginalized in typical health professions training programs.

Academic medicine must play a major part in training clinicians for the new roles of providers called for by integrative approaches, including the need to promote research to test the effectiveness of new practice models. Evidence of the benefits of the integrated, patient-oriented approach can be found in another neglected realm of medical education, palliative care, which in the face of terminal illness focuses on whole person needs, addresses social and family issues, and promotes compassion and healing, even though cure is impossible. But, while academic medicine has been a constant source of innovations in specialty care, few medical schools and training institutions have become engaged in approaches to improving general clinical care or development of provider models to improve care delivery.

Some elements of an integrated approach to health care also have their roots in practices that began under the rubric of complementary and alternative medicine (CAM). The effectiveness of such approaches has been strengthened as experience and evidence has been gained. In 2003–2004, the National Center for Complementary and Alternative Medicine sponsored a series of grants to strengthen awareness and knowledge about complementary and alternative medicine practices among medical students. The goal was to broaden the array of evidence-based techniques that physicians have at their disposal. A common finding from these projects was that culture change, including faculty development, was a necessary accompaniment to curriculum changes, and the result is a growing presence of relevant courses in the nursing and medical curricula. Expansion of these trends requires additional research, resources, incentives, continuing education courses, licensure requirements, and, perhaps, ultimately, reimbursement incentives.

A number of academic centers are beginning to change, adding formal integrative medicine programs, including research, education, and clinical care components to speed the transformation toward more integrated, coordinated care management. Others, mindful of the deep interest of many patients and providers in CAM practices—ranging from the use of mindfulness meditation, acupuncture, massage and biofeedback, to nutritional practices and dietary supplements (e.g., herbs, vitamins, minerals)—have developed research, education, and practice programs that seek to deepen the evidence base, in order to accelerate the application of effective health care practices. Many medical and nursing faculty and students are philosophically supportive of greater integration of conventional and CAM therapies but referral to these modalities is infrequent as a result not only of limitations in the evidence base but also of prevailing professional attitudes and beliefs.

Progress in evidence-based integrative care therefore depends on leadership from academic health professions schools to develop the interdisciplinary research and training programs. New models for residency training programs, such as the "Integrative Family Medicine" pilot program, conducted at six pilot sites[2] around the country that combine family medicine residencies and integrative fellowships appear promising. These new models could be especially effective if paired with incentives for academic health centers through research funds, with accreditation and reimbursement programs, and with incentives for practitioners through licensure and board certification examinations.

Take the example of prospective medicine as a component of an integrated approach to health care. For prospective medicine to be central to medical education would require changes in basic sciences teaching, clinical education, and medical school culture. The basic sciences would need to include teaching about the role of predictive biomarkers, the evolution from health to disease, and the points of potential intervention along that continuum. Clinical education should include practice in conducting comprehensive medical evaluations, health planning, establishing good two-way patient communication and motivation, and disease management.

These improvements depend on fundamentally altering health professions training to focus on interdisciplinary education and practical experience in working in effective care teams that can reduce medical errors, improve health care quality, and put at clinicians' disposal the full array of skills needed for effective patient care and wellness promotion. Teams are essential for the best care of people with chronic illnesses,

---

[2]University of Arizona, Beth Israel/Albert Einstein College of Medicine (New York, N.Y.), Maine Medical Center, Middlesex Hospital (Middletown, Conn.), Oregon Health & Science University, and the University of Wisconsin.

although impending shortages in primary care physicians and other team members will increasingly hamper team-based practice. This, too, requires basic changes in the structure of economic incentives to emphasize primary care and health outcomes (Bodenheimer et al., 2009).

PUBLIC AND PATIENT COMMUNICATION STRATEGIES

Increasing public support for a radical change in the current fragmented system of medical care is reflected in the growth of advocacy groups that support health care that centers on the patient, with all the attendant changes implied. A long-term goal of many such groups is to influence health policy to remove regulatory and reimbursement barriers to preventive care and to support personalized medicine research. These groups sponsor educational sessions to acquaint the public and policy makers with integrative medicine concepts.

People who support these changes in the health care system and who seek out and use integrative medicine practices are generally self-directed and more interested in taking a greater role in their own health care. They typically want more of a conversation with their physicians, which can be brief yet still extremely effective, that produces shared expectations and a treatment plan that both sides buy into. The one-way stream of information to which patients are usually subjected has been notably ineffective in encouraging adherence to treatment plans. Greater patient involvement and physician listening might result in plans more relevant to patients' circumstances and, therefore, improve adherence rates.

Perhaps the lack of two-way dialogue has contributed to an inclination among growing numbers of people to seek complementary and alternative medical practices over which they have direct control. About half of healthy individuals report using one or more of these modalities in an attempt to enhance or maintain health and functioning. Ironically, this can exacerbate the divide between patients and providers. Patients often worry that their physicians would disapprove of some of their CAM practices, they frequently avoid mentioning them—a potentially harmful outcome if an alternative practice interferes with medical treatment. For example, a study of cardiac surgery patients found that about 70 percent used some form of complementary therapy. Most commonly, patients used vitamins (54 percent), prayer (36 percent), nutritional therapy (17 percent), massage, herbs, chiropractic services, and meditation

(10 to 11 percent each). Only one in five patients discussed these practices with their surgeons. Unfortunately, 45 percent of the patients were using a therapy, especially certain herbs, that could negatively affect the results of their surgery (Oz, 2004).

Recognizing that patients are very likely using these modalities, strategies for improving communication between physicians and patients about CAM are important. Additional research is needed on the clinical effectiveness of CAM, and using the clinical environment to implement carefully planned research protocols may further enhance clinicians' familiarity with them, while fostering greater trust between clinicians and patients.

Good patient–physician communication also is important to integrative medicine in a much wider sense. It is essential to changing individual attitudes, beliefs, and practices of patients and health systems alike. Practitioners need the ability to emotionally and intellectually convince patients that change in their lifestyle or health care practices is required and to use intellectual and economic arguments to convince health care institutions and systems that a better style of practice will benefit them, too.

Patients in general want better communication with their providers. Whatever they feel about the health system, they trust their own physicians and believe they provide high-quality care. A recent Kaiser Permanente study of enrollees found that they judged the quality of care provided by the system almost solely on these relationships. Providers and payers alike have a greater responsibility than previously acknowledged to nurture those relationships, for several reasons: growing awareness that satisfaction with the health system improves health care outcomes; from an economic standpoint, it also may reduce patient churn; and, knowing enrollees are likely to stay in a health system or insurance plan for a longer period greatly increases insurers' incentives to work on disease prevention and wellness.

RESEARCH CONTEXT AND PRIORITIES

Advances in the research base have revealed the promise of integrative medicine and will be key to its progress. As a result of contributions from research in epidemiology, genetics, endocrinology, psychology, and health services, the core knowledge needed to shift the practice of medicine to a more integrated model—emphasizing personalized, predictive, preventive, and participatory approaches—is now available. A much stronger science base provides the foundation for knowing about the important elements of prevention and health promotion, about the importance of exercise and dietary factors on health prospects, about individual predispositions to disease and disability, about the effect of stress and psychologically supportive factors on disease processes, about the interrelationships between the neurologic and endocrine systems, and about the harm done by discontinuities in care. We are now in a position for contemporary science to help understand health insights and practices that sometimes span the course of recorded history.

Yet our established knowledge is still young. When patients have multiple chronic conditions, the ability to manage, monitor, slow disease progress, and avoid complications becomes increasingly complex, and research is needed on ways to optimize and balance treatment choices for individual patients. Many chronic conditions—even normal aging—are frequently accompanied by psychological symptoms that affect patients' ability to recover from illness and motivation to maintain health. These complicated situations emphasize the need for health services research to identify and develop practice models that facilitate delivery of integrated, patient-centered care, including ways to better incorporate mental health services into ordinary clinical practice. High-profile research into these questions also will enhance the stature of primary care in medical schools, where prestige is heavily based on research capacity and achievement.

In the past few years, research projects by government agencies, industry, and academic institutions have "begun to provide an increasingly rich infrastructure to identify the mechanisms involved in transitioning from health to disease and the biomarkers . . . (that) predict clinical events" (Snyderman and Yoediono, 2008). Knowledge derived from the Human Genome Project, the International HapMap Project, and growing information from the fields of genomics, proteomics, metabolomics, bioinformatics, medical technologies, and systems biology are making this transition possible.

Increasingly, researchers and practitioners are able to use biomarkers to predict and track disease and assess the effects of treatment. A national interest in personalized health care is focused on combining genomic research breakthroughs with improved health information technology to enable susceptibilities to be identified as early as possible, so that clinicians can take and recommend preventive countermeasures. Prospects are developing for biomarkers to help predict the onset or course of some breast and prostate cancers, as well as appropriate dosages of certain medications. Used in combination with traditional clinical prognostic tools, the new predictive technologies will create a sound scientific base for many new preventive approaches.

The temptation may exist for clinicians (and some patients, too) to treat genomics, proteomics, and so on as the next generation of high-tech tools that provide quick answers to clinical problems. However, such advances will never substitute for clinicians' and patients' judgments, and the data derived from these tools should be seen as an opportunity to build a long-term relationship focused on health maintenance. The data provide a more accurate long-range forecast of outcomes, which enables clinicians and patients to set in motion long-term strategies to minimize identified risks through close monitoring and the management of related behavioral and environmental factors. Used appropriately, these technologies should foster closer patient–physician collaboration, not curtail it.

Priorities and challenges for research in integrative medicine start with the most fundamental concepts. People from different cultures vary in their understanding and views of the origins of disease. In our culture, biological processes are almost always considered the sole culprit in an illness, with occasional reference to the effect of psychosocial factors on disease processes. Some other cultures, for example, attribute disease to malevolent spirits or supernatural forces. In the multicultural U.S. society, the very different lenses through which physicians see the world, on one hand, and the traditions and beliefs of various cultural groups, on the other, lead to widely disparate world views, misunderstanding, and counterproductive communication on matters vital to the effectiveness of treatment (Fadiman, 1997). Researchers, as much as clinicians, are challenged to take these vastly different perspectives into account when assessing patient outcomes.

A key challenge to research therefore lies not only in developing the biological, molecular, and advanced imaging tools for predicting and early identification of disease, but also in applying these tools to improve the process of care and support the interactive and integrative nature of the care experience, including:

- improved strategies for patient engagement, through education, communication, motivation, and support;
- identifying lessons from related disciplines, such as palliative care, stress management, and social connectedness;

- epidemiologic studies that address patient and cost outcomes across populations of different races, ethnicities, and socioeconomic status;
- evaluating alternative professional education programs;
- developing and testing new health service delivery models and evaluating the effectiveness and cost-effectiveness of practice-based integrative care; and
- assessing the impact of alternative reimbursement policies, regulations, and incentives on the adoption of integrative medicine principles.

ECONOMICS AND POLICY

Coursing throughout all dimensions of health care that is integrative in nature—care that integrates prevention and treatment, mind and body, the traditional and the emerging, the elements and stages of the care experience—is the need to align economic incentives appropriately. This is a matter of necessity not simply for care that is more effective but for care that is more efficient as well.

The nation is now confronting an economic crisis unlike any in nearly a century—and perhaps ever. With U.S. health care costs, already so much higher than elsewhere and still rising, making our industries less profitable and less internationally competitive, and with the health system underperforming at such a significant level, it is already a substantial part of our nation's near-term economic problem. But, without dramatic change, it is destined to become a much larger share in the future. Although much more work needs to be done to provide the economic models and proof of the return on investment that an integrated health care system could provide, both common sense and the studies in hand support the precept that preventing disease and injury is preferable to attempting rescue after the damage is done—preferable in terms of patient outcomes and quality of life, cost savings, and increased economic productivity. Further, evidence to date suggests that adequate economic incentives can motivate clinicians and institutions to change their practices toward a more integrated model of care.

Well-designed educational efforts to inform patients about their care options have been shown to influence patients' choice of therapies, and they frequently choose less aggressive treatments, including surgery, than their physicians would have recommended (Wennberg et al., 2007).

Preventive and disease management programs supported by employers for their workers have been shown to improve productivity and reduce costs. A Duke University study showed that a proactive management program for patients with congestive heart failure could improve health outcomes *and* reduce health care costs.

Because most economic studies done to date have not been able to adequately capture in economic terms the full range of benefits that accrue to keeping people healthier and happier, some payers take only the short-term view. They limit integrative services because they see only near-term costs and fear increases in demand. In fact, when these services are covered, use may rise, but the few studies that address costs suggest that greater use may not increase overall expenditures; rather, it can reduce costs by serving as a lower-cost, lower-tech substitution for later needs.

Current payment and reimbursement incentives militate against development of clinical care models that use an integrative medicine approach. The procedure-centered, acute-care orientation of U.S. payers is in stark contrast to the more whole-patient-centered, prevention-oriented philosophy in some other countries. However, a small, but growing number of U.S. physician practices to varying degrees have adopted an integrated medicine style of practice. They put more emphasis on teamwork, better meld physical and mental health services, rely more heavily on nonphysician practitioners for patient education and counseling, involve complementary and alternative medicine practices and practitioners as needed, implement electronic health records, and organize their practices in other ways to make care more wellness oriented. Some of these physician practices have been found to not only increase and maintain patients' health more effectively than traditional approaches, but also to reduce health care costs. Reimbursement strategies that support this kind of practice, especially its counseling and educational elements, or share payers' savings with the practice will be essential for widespread adoption.

REFERENCES

Bodenheimer, T., E. Chen, and H. D. Bennett. 2009. Confronting the growing burden of chronic disease: Can the U.S. health care workforce do the job? *Health Affairs* 28:64-74.

Fadiman, A. 1997. *The spirit catches you and you fall down.* New York: Farrar, Straus, & Giroux.

IOM (Institute of Medicine). 2001. *Crossing the Quality Chasm: A New Health System for the 21st Century.* Washington, DC: National Academy Press.

McGinnis, J. M., and W. H. Foege. 1993. Actual causes of death in the United States. *Journal of the American Medical Association* 270:2207-2212.

Oz, M. 2004. Emerging role of integrative medicine in cardiovascular disease. *Cardiology in Review* 12:120-123.

Snyderman, R., and Z. Yoediono. 2008. *Academic Medicine* 83:707-714.

Wennberg, J. E., A. M. O'Connor, E. D. Collins, and J. N. Weinstein. 2007. Extending the p4p agenda, part 1: How Medicare can improve patient decision making and reduce unnecessary care. *Health Affairs* 26(6):1564-1574.